Benjamin KASIWA

Study on the needs for the establishment of homes for the elderly

Benjamin KASIWA

Study on the needs for the establishment of homes for the elderly

Study on the needs of third age people

ScienciaScripts

Imprint
Any brand names and product names mentioned in this book are subject to trademark, brand or patent protection and are trademarks or registered trademarks of their respective holders. The use of brand names, product names, common names, trade names, product descriptions etc. even without a particular marking in this work is in no way to be construed to mean that such names may be regarded as unrestricted in respect of trademark and brand protection legislation and could thus be used by anyone.

Cover image: www.ingimage.com

This book is a translation from the original published under ISBN 978-613-1-58940-9.

Publisher:
Sciencia Scripts
is a trademark of
Dodo Books Indian Ocean Ltd. and OmniScriptum S.R.L publishing group

120 High Road, East Finchley, London, N2 9ED, United Kingdom
Str. Armeneasca 28/1, office 1, Chisinau MD-2012, Republic of Moldova, Europe
Managing Directors: Ieva Konstantinova, Victoria Ursu
info@omniscriptum.com

Printed at: see last page
ISBN: 978-620-3-64314-5

Copyright © Benjamin KASIWA
Copyright © 2021 Dodo Books Indian Ocean Ltd. and OmniScriptum S.R.L publishing group

TABLE OF CONTENTS

Chapter 1	13
Chapter 2	25
Chapter 3	41
Chapter 4	48
Chapter 5	70
Chapter 6	78

EPIGRAPH

"In Africa, if an old man dies, it is like a library burning.

Words of Amadou Hampaté Bâ.

SUMMARY

The present study is about "Study on the needs of the establishment of homes for the elderly experienced by the elderly in the health zone of Goma", we wanted to know what are the needs of the establishment of homes for the elderly experienced by the elderly in the health zone of Goma. From this important constant, three specific questions followed:

> What are the housing conditions for the elderly in the Goma health zone?
> What are the housing needs of the elderly in the Goma health zone?
> What are the types of housing orientations expressed by the elderly in the Goma health zone?

Based on these questions we have formulated the following anticipated answers:

S Food insecurity, psycho-physical abuse, lack of respect within their families, low financial contribution would be the conditions of accommodation of the elderly in the health zone of Goma;

S Premises adapted to their physical conditions, the desire to live in the home, the need to protect their integuments would be housing needs experienced by the elderly in the health zone of Goma;

S Social assistance, family assistance, psychological support, medical care, economic assistance through IGAs would be the types of orientations expressed by the elderly in terms of housing in the health zone of Goma.

In the search for an answer to these questions, we set ourselves the general objective of evaluating the needs of the establishment of homes for the elderly experienced by the elderly in the health zone of Goma. The pursuit of this objective led us to operationalize it in four specific objectives

> Determine the housing conditions for the elderly in the health zone of Goma;
> Identify the housing needs experienced by the elderly in the health zone of Goma;
> Determine the types of housing orientations expressed by the elderly in the Goma health zone.

This study is both evaluative and cross-sectional, and used both quantitative and qualitative data. The sample size for this study consisted of 141 older adults who fall within the age range of 65 to 84 years and older. The data was collected by means of a survey questionnaire administered to 141 elderly people. It was also necessary to use an unstructured interview technique with a supporting interview guide to facilitate the collection of qualitative information from three household heads in the Goma health zone. Quantitative data were processed and analyzed in Microsoft Word and SPSS (Statistical Package of Social Sciences) software under Windows, and qualitative data were analyzed manually to test the hypotheses and arrive at the final results. After analyzing, processing, analyzing and interpreting the data, we reached the following conclusions:

In observing the housing conditions of the ^{elderly} in the Goma health zone, the results of this study show that more than half, i.e., 57.5% of the subjects live in good housing conditions, 26.3% say that the conditions are fairly good, and a minority say that they live in poor conditions. Similarly, those who live in very good conditions represent 3.5%. A very low proportion of 2.1% and 1.4% of respondents say that they live in very bad and poor accommodation conditions. Speaking of the type of food, only 37.6% of respondents eat cassava and corn, 24.1% eat vegetables and fruits, those who usually eat beans and rice represent 15.6% against 13.5% who eat fish. Similarly, a minority, 7.8%, eat whatever they can find. This leads us to say that the elderly in the Goma Health Zone are more accustomed to taking protective foods. From these results, it is indicated that almost half (46.8%) eat twice a day followed by 25.5% who eat three times a day. Those who eat more than three times a day represent a proportion of 14.2% compared to those who eat once a day who occupy a proportion of 12.8% and finally an old man or 0.7% who said that he eats according to the availability of food. Concerning the types of abuse suffered by the elderly within their families or elsewhere, the results of this study show that 85 respondents (60.3%) denied that they had ever suffered physical abuse within their families or elsewhere, compared to 56 respondents (39.7%) who said that they had already suffered this act of physical abuse. In the same study, 89 respondents, or more than half (63.1%), said they had already been subjected to psychological abuse within their respective families or elsewhere, compared to 52 respondents (36.9%) who denied having ever been subjected to psychological abuse.

With regard to decision-making within the family, the study shows that the majority of respondents (72.3%) said that they were consulted during care within their respective families, compared to 27.7% who denied or said the opposite. If we look at the results of the score table, we see that out of **141** elderly people in the Goma health zone, **88** respondents **(62.4%)** answered positively to the criteria of good housing conditions, while **53** respondents **(37.6%)** indicated that the conditions were poor. Based on the above scores, we can conclude that the housing conditions for the elderly in the Goma Health Zone are ***good.*** This has led us to invalidate the first hypothesis that food insecurity, psycho-physical abuse, low esteem within their families, and low financial contribution would be the housing conditions of the elderly in the Goma health zone.

If we consider the housing needs experienced by the elderly in the Goma health zone, the results of this study show that out of a total of 141 respondents, more than half (58%) live in a house made of durable materials, followed by those who live in houses made of planks (54.6%) and a minority (2.8% and 1.4%) who live in houses made of tarpaulin and straw. Similarly, it appears that more than half, i.e. 53.9% of the respondents, say that the house they live in allows them to exercise all the physical movement against 46.1% who say the opposite. In the same way, more than half, that is to say 63,8%, affirm that their dwellings are served with drinking water and electricity whereas 36,2% prove an opposite opinion. The results of the same study show that more than half, 57.4%, say that they want to live in the home, while 42.6% do not want to for the rest of their lives. If we look at the results of the score table, we see that out of **141** elderly people in the Goma health zone, **76** respondents **(54%)** answered positively to the criteria of good housing conditions, while **65** respondents **(46%)** indicated that the housing conditions were poor. Based on the above scores, we can conclude that the housing conditions of the elderly in the Goma Health Zone are *quite good.* This led us to assert the second hypothesis according to which the premises adapted to their physical conditions, the desire to live in the home, and the need to protect their integuments would be housing needs experienced by the third age people in the Goma health zone.

Based on the types of orientations expressed by the elderly in terms of housing in the health zone of Goma, the results of this study show that more than half, 53.9%, have already benefited from external social assistance, as opposed to 46.1% who, in their turn, have benefited from the services of a social worker.

have never benefited from it. Regarding family support, the present study shows that a large proportion (94.3%) of respondents wish to have support from their respective families against a minority (5.7%) who do not. Concerning the suffering of an illness, it appears from this study that a large majority (97.2%) have already suffered from an illness during their daily life against a minority (2.3%) who say they have never suffered from an illness. For those who said they had ever suffered from an illness, more than half (59.8%) had resorted to hospital treatment, 38% had resorted to self-medication and the use of medical plants, while 2.2% relied solely on prayer. However, a large majority (93.6%) of the respondents wanted specialized medical assistance in case of illness, while a minority (6.4%) did not. If we consider the results from the score table, which show that out of **141** elderly people in the Goma health zone, **103** respondents (**73%**) answered favorably to the criteria for the types of referrals that are good, while **38** respondents (**27%**) revealed the opposite. Based on the above scores, we can conclude that the types of referrals among the elderly in the Goma Health Zone are *good and they want to stay in the home for the rest of their lives.* This allowed us to affirm the third hypothesis according to which social assistance, family assistance, psychological support, medical care, and economic assistance through IGAs would be the types of orientations expressed by the [third] age people in terms of housing in the Goma health zone.

Taking into account the results and conclusions of this work, we suggest the following:

To the government
> That it strengthens the social security system throughout the national territory and gives all former workers in both the private and public sectors access to a pension;
> That it supports the organizations and associations that have in their midst initiatives of care or support of any kind for the elderly.

To the person in charge of the elderly in the health zone of Goma
> That they respond to the needs of economic, social, medical and health assistance.

To future researchers

Whether they continue to address issues with the same constituency as ours or even approach this issue from the perspective of a feasibility study for setting up a home or

We hope that we have set a milestone and opened a great breach in a great construction site which is research in order to build a huge edifice which is science.

EXECUTIVE SUMMARRY

The present survey is about l' "Survey on the needs of the setting up of the homes of the old men felt by people of 3rd age in the zone of health of Goma", we wanted to know what are the needs of the setting up of the homes of the old men felt by people of 3rd age in the zone of health of Goma. Of this constant important, had ensued here three specific questions - under:

> What are the conditions of lodging of 3rd age people in the zone of health of Goma?
> What are the needs in lodging felt by people of 3rd age in the zone of health of Goma?
> What are the types of orientations expressed by people of 3rd age concerning lodging in the zone of health of Goma?

Leaving from these questions us formulated the answers anticipated following:

- S The food insecurity, the maltraitances psychophysiques, the déconsidération within their family, weak financial contribution would be conditions of lodging of 3rd age people in the zone of health of Goma;
- S The local adapted to their physical conditions, the wish to live in the home, the needs to protect their teguments would be needs in lodging felt by people of 3rd age in the zone of health of Goma;
- S The social aid, the domestic helps, the psychological accompaniment, taken in medical charge, economic aid by the AGR would be the types of orientations expressed by people of 3rd age concerning lodging in the zone of health of Goma.

In the research of an answer to these questionnements, we assigned ourselves to reach the general objective to identify the needs of the setting up of the homes of the old men felt by people of 3rd age in the zone of health of Goma. The pursuit of the realization of this objective pushed us to the opérationnaliser in four following specific objectives:

> To determine the conditions of lodging of 3rd age people in the zone of health of Goma ;
> To identify the needs in lodging felt by people of 3rd age in the zone of health of Goma;
> To determine the types of orientations expressed by people of 3rd age concerning lodging in the zone of health of Goma.

The present survey is at a time évaluative and transversal, and made call to quantitative and qualitative data. The size of the sample of this survey was composed of 141 old men who are located in the age group understood between 65 years and 84 years and more. The data have been harvested with the help of a questionnaire of investigation managed by hundred forty one old men. But also, he/it was necessary to us to resort to a technique of interview non structured with a guide of interview to the support to facilitate the collection of the qualitative information by three persons responsible of households of the zone of health of Goma. Thus, the quantitative data have been treated and have been analyzed in the software Microsoft Word and SPSS (Statistical Package of Social Sciences) under Windows and those that are qualitative have been analyzed by hand in the goal to verify the hypotheses and to arrive to the final results. After analysis, treatment, spoliation and interpretation of the data, we succeeded to the following findings:

While observing the conditions of lodging of 3rd age people in the zone of health of Goma, he/it is evident from results of this survey that more of half are 57,5% of the topics live in conditions of good lodging, 26,3% say that the conditions are good enough against a minority is that appreciates a bad manner. In the same way, those that live in very good conditions represent 3,5%. A proportion very bass of 2,1% and 1,4% of them investigated say that they live in conditions of very bad and mediocre lodging. Speaking of the type of food, he/it comes out again than on the whole of them investigated, only 37,6% take the foufou of cassava and corn, 24,1% eat the vegetables and the fruits, those that have the habit to take bean and rice represent 15,6% against 13,5% that take fish. In the same way, a minority is 7,8% take everything that they find. It brings us to say that the old men of the zone of health of Goma have the habit more to take the protective food. Departure these results he/it is indicated that close to half is 46,8% take the meal two times per consistent day of 25,5% that make it three times per day. Those that take more than three times per day represent a proportion of 14,2% in relation to those that make it once per day that occupy a proportion of 12,8% and in end an old man is 0.7% that said that he eats according to the availability of food. Concerning the types of maltraitances undergone by the old men within their family or elsewhere, the results of this survey show that 85 investigated either 60,3% deny that them not undergone a physical maltraitance ever to their consideration within their respective families or elsewhere against 56 investigated either 39,7% that affirm to have undergone this physical maltraitance act already. Of this same survey, 89 investigated either more of half are 63,1% affirm to have undergone a psychological maltraitance already to their consideration within their respective families or elsewhere against 52 investigated either 36,9% that deny to have undergone a psychological maltraitance already. Being about the decision making within the family, he/it ensues of this survey that the majority is 72,3% of the respondents affirm have been consulted at the time of the hold in charge within their respective families against 27,7% that deny or that say the opposite. If we consider the results descended of score picture that raise that, on a strength of 141 old men of the zone of health of Goma, 88 investigated either 62,4% of the respondents answered the criterias of the lodging conditions that are good favorably, whereas a strength of 53 investigated either 37,6% revealed us that these last are bad. On basis of these evoked above scores, we can conclude while saying that the conditions of lodging at people of third ages within Zone of health of Goma are good. It brought us to invalidate the first hypothesis according to which the food insecurity, the maltraitances psychophysiques, the déconsidération within their family, weak financial contribution would be conditions of lodging of 3rd age people in the zone of health of Goma.

If we consider the needs in lodging felt by people of 3rd age in the zone of health of Goma, the results of this survey show that on a strength of 141 investigated, more of half are 58% accommodate a dwelling in lasting material followed of those that lodge in houses in board is 54,6% against a minority is 2,8% and 1,4% that accommodate some houses in awning and in straw. In the same way, he/it comes out again that more of half are 53,9% of them investigated the house that they live in their permit to exercise all change physics against 46,1% that say the opposite. In the same way, more of half are 63,8% affirm that their lodgings are gone against in drinking water and in electricity whereas 36,2% prove a contrary opinion. The results of this same survey show that, more of half are 57,4% say that they have the wish to live in the home, while 42,6% don't wish it for the rest of life. If we consider the results descended of score picture raise that, on a strength of 141 old men of the zone of health of Goma, 76 investigated either 54% of the respondents answered the criterias of the lodging conditions that are good favorably, whereas a strength of 65 investigated either 46% revealed us that these last are bad. On basis of these evoked above scores, we can conclude while saying that the conditions of lodging at people of third ages within Zone of health of Goma are good enough. It brought us to affirm the second hypothesis according to which the local adapted to their physical conditions, the wish to live in the home, the needs to protect their teguments would be needs in lodging felt by people of 3rd age in the zone of health of Goma.

Leaving from the types of orientations expressed by people of 3rd age concerning lodging in the zone of health of Goma, the results of this survey show that more of half are 53,9% benefitted an outside social aid already against 46,1% that never benefitted some from their tower. Being about the helps descended of the family, the present survey shows that a big proportion is 94,3% of respondents have the wish to have a help descended of their respective families against a minority is 5,7% that don't want it. Concerning the suffering of an illness, he/it is evident from this survey that a big majority is 97,2% endured an illness already during their daily life against a minority is 2,3% that say that they never suffered from an illness. For those that affirmed to have suffered already from an illness, more of half are 59,8% made resort to the of the hospital, 38% made resort to the self-medication and the use of the medical plants whereas 2,2% don't trust the prayer only. However, a big majority is 93,6% of them investigated wish a medical aid specialized in case of illness against a minority is 6,4% of contrary opinion. If we consider the results descended of the score picture raise that, on a strength of 141 old men of the zone of health of Goma, 103 investigated either a majority (73%) some respondents answered the criterias of the types of orientations that are good favorably, whereas a strength of 38 investigated either 27% revealed us that the opposite. On basis of these evoked above scores, we can conclude while saying that the types of orientations at people of third ages within Zone of health of Goma are good and wish to be lodged in the home remained it of their life. It allowed us to affirm the third hypothesis according to which social Aid, the domestic helps, the psychological accompaniment, taken in medical charge, economic aid by the AGR would be the types of orientations expressed by people of 3rd age concerning lodging in the zone of health of Goma.

Holding in account the results and the findings given out in this work, we suggest what follows: **To the government**

> That he/it reinforces the system of social security in all the extent of the national territory and makes reach all ex-workers so much the private sector that of the public sector to one retirement;

> That he/it sustains the organizations and associations that have in their breast of the hold initiatives in load or any support to people of third age.

To the person responsible old men of the zone of health of Goma

> That they answer the needs as well in economic aid, social and medical or sanitary aid.

To the future researchers

> That they continue to approach the topics having the same circumscription that ours or even to approach this question under the angle of a survey of feasibility of setting up of a home or retirement homes, thing that we didn't make; because we hope to have put the pole and opened a big breach in a big yard that is research in order to construct an immense building that is the science.

ACRONYMS AND ABBREVIATIONS

- **AGR**   Income-generating activity
- **AS**   : Health Area;
- **BCZ**   Central Office of the Health Zone;
- **C to d**   : That is;
- **CEPAC**   Community of Pentecostal Churches in Central Africa;
- **COGE**   : Management Committee;
- **AOC**   : Health Committee;
- **CS**   : Health Center;
- **EDS-EDC** : Demographic and Health Survey;
- **FSDC**   : Faculty of Community Health and Development ;
- **HGR**   : General Referral Hospital;
- **INSS**   National Institute of Social Security,
- **IT**   : Nurse Attending;
- **WHO**   World Health Organization;
- **NGO**   : Non-Governmental Organization ;
- **PVD**   : Sending country of development ;
- **DRC**   Democratic Republic of Congo;
- **VAR**   : Airway regulation;
- **SNEL**   : National Electricity Company
- **ULPGL**   : Université Libre des Pays des Grands lacs ;
- **USD**   United States Dollars;
- **WHO**   : World Health Organization;
- **ZS**   : Health Zone.

Chapter One.
GENERAL INTRODUCTION
1.1. General information about the research
1.1.1. Introduction to the study

The aging of the world's population in both developing and developed countries is an indicator of improving global health. The global population aged 60 and over has doubled since 1980 and is expected to reach two billion by 2050. This is a cause for celebration. Older people make important contributions to society as family members, volunteers, and labor force participants. With the wisdom they have acquired throughout their lives, they are a vital social resource. However, with these positives also come unprecedented health challenges for the 21st century. [1]

The care of the elderly is an issue of concern in the world, despite the efforts made in developed countries to date, the indicators are still alarming. It is important to prepare caregivers and societies to meet the special needs of older populations. This includes training health professionals in geriatrics; preventing and treating age-related chronic diseases; designing sustainable policies for long-term care and palliative care; and developing services and environments that are age-friendly. KARSTEN Thormaehlen, says, *"The sooner we act, the more likely we are to make this global transformation work for everyone. Countries that invest in healthy aging can expect significant social and economic benefits for the entire community.* [2]

1.1.2. General information on the study environment
1.1.2.1. History of the Goma Health Zone

The creation of the Goma health area dates back to 1985. It was around the year 2000 that the city was divided into two health areas, NDOSHO and KIZIBA. In the KATOYI health area, the Berthes health center was opened. In total, the URBANO-rural health zone had a general hospital of reference, two hospital centers, 18 health centers (HGR/Goma, CH CBK: Virunga, CH. By his letter n°251/IPS-NK/449/2003, the Provincial Health Inspector of North Kivu proposed to the Ministry of Health to divide the URBANO-rural health zone of Goma into 3 health zones. [3]

In mid-October 2003, a division workshop was organized at the KARIBU hotel for the harmonization and validation of the health map of North Kivu during the Congolese gathering by the DRC in the middle of the rebellion. The division will be effective on the decree of the Ministry of Public Health in DRC n°12520/CAB/MIN/AF/O89/2003 of November 11, 2003 defining the health map of the province of North Kivu divided into 34 health zones. The URBANO-rural health zone of Goma was divided into 2 health zones within the administrative boundaries of the communes of Goma and KARISIMBI:

- Urban health zone of Goma: 139489 inhabitants

---

[1] KARSTENThormaehlen, *aging and quality of life*, Ghana, 2012, available at http://www.who.int/features/factfiles/ageing/fr/, accessed March 22, 2014 at 9:20 am.
[2] Same as
[3] *Goma* health zone central office, *annual report*, 2012-2013, p13.

- Urban health zone of KARISIMBI : 340426 inhabitants

After the division, the urban health zone of Goma functions with the HGR Goma, Charité maternelle, CS CASOP, KATINDO, HIMBI, Carmel, KYESHERO, Centre Chrétien du Lac Kivu (CCLK) and BUHIMBA. [4]

1. 1.2.2. Geographic location

The Goma health zone is located in the DRC, province of North Kivu, city of Goma, commune of Goma. It has a surface area of 150Km2 and is limited:

> In the East by the Republic of Rwanda
> To the West by the health zone of KIROTSHE
> In the North by the health zone of KARISIMBI
> In the South by the lake Kivu

---

[4] Same as

I.1.2.3 Demographic situation

The Goma health zone has a population of 180364 inhabitants in 2012 and 185775 inhabitants in 2013 distributed in 9 health areas. This population is growing due to the phenomenon of rural exodus and the persistence of insecurity in the region.

Tableau 1: Demographic character of the Goma health zone by health area [5]

Health areas	Total population 2012	Total population 2013
CASOP	11719	12071
MAPENDO	57690	59521
HIMBI	13246	13643
KATINDO	14804	15248
HEAL AFRICA	8432	8685
CARMEL	17015	17525
KYESHERO	36766	37869
CCLK	14534	14970
BUHIMBA	6158	6343
TOTAL	180364	185775

From this total population, the health zone of Goma has within it a total of 19586 people of the third ages (55 to 85 years and more) for the year 2013. These people are distributed or found in the different neighborhoods of the Goma commune, as is the case in the Goma zone.

Tableau 2: Synoptic table of the population of the 3rd age in the health zone of Goma [6]

Age range	Men	Women	Total
55-59 years old	3805	3085	6890
60-64 years old	2468	2167	4635
65-69 years old	1375	2545	3920
70-74 years old	764	1016	1780
75-79 years old	546	738	1284
80-84 years old	300	454	753
85 years and older	188	136	324
Total	9446	10141	19586

It should be noted that as the WHO says that the age range of the elderly begins at 65 years, for us, the number of elderly people from 65 to 85 years and more is 8061 elderly people in the health zone of Goma. [7]

1.1.2.4. Health situation

The health zone of Goma is made up of 9 health areas, each health area is represented by a health center. In addition to these health centers, the Goma health zone contains a general reference hospital "Charité maternelle", the provincial general hospital of North Kivu, numerous hospital centers: Heal Africa, Bethesda (CBKN Ndosho), 8th CEPAC/Kyeshero, Docs, numerous medical centers, CEDIGO, Belle vue, Camellias, adventist center, CIMAK and many private health posts.

---

[5] Central Office of the *Goma* Health Zone, *annual report*, op cit
[6] Bureau de l'état civil, commune de Goma, census report by age group, 2013
[7] Id.

The health zone of Goma also has many traditional treatment houses where traditional practitioners are present. [8]

1.1.2.5. Environmental situation

The Goma health zone is located on the shores of Lake Kivu and occupies the southern part of the Goma-SAKE road. All the health areas are reforested with natural trees and fruit trees in some concessions. In the Goma health zone, there are some green spaces: BUHIMBA, ULPGL, RVA and Mount Goma to purify the air. The Goma health zone covers the wealthy neighborhoods of the city of Goma: Volcanoes (city), Katindo left, HIMBI, KYESHERO. It is electrified by the SNEL but sometimes experiences power cuts. The population obtains its water from the tap, from REGIDESO, from the lake and from rainwater.

1.1.2.6. Educational situation

There are several kindergartens, primary, secondary and vocational schools, higher institutions, state and private universities.

1.1.2.7. Socio-cultural situation

The health zone of Goma was a reception zone during the last volcanic eruption (2002) and following the insecurity in the surroundings of Goma (Masisi, Walikale, Bukavu). The rural exodus has led to an increase in the population, which is cosmopolitan. The population is cosmopolitan. It is made up of Shi, Nande, Rega, Hunde, Nyanga, Havu, Hutu, Tutsi and other tribes of the DRC, including foreigners. The official language is Swahili as well as vernacular languages according to the tribes. This cosmopolitan population is divided into several religious denominations: Catholics, Protestants, revivalist churches, Adventists, Jehovah's Witnesses, Baha'i Faith, Muslims... [9].

It should be noted that the Goma health zone, with a very high number of elderly people, has no home for the elderly, no retirement home, and no center for the care of elderly people. This situation has existed since the creation of this zone, so there has never been a home for the elderly in the Goma health zone.

1.1.2.8. Economic situation

Most of the population in the Goma health zone is employed (working) in several state, private and humanitarian sectors. They include government services, local, national and international NGOs, banks, savings and loan cooperatives, telecommunication institutions, stores, stores, travel agencies (land, air, river), photo studios, gas stations, hotels, bistros, markets, public phones, hair salons, public secretariats, cyber cafes, food stores, garages, sewing shops, carpentry shops, hardware stores, and bakeries [10]

---

[8] Central Office of the *Goma* Health Zone, *annual report*, op cit
[9] Same as
[10] Central Office of the *Goma* Health Zone, *annual report*, op cit

1.2. Issue

Since the 1st World Assembly on Ageing in 1982, the world has undergone a great demographic change. In the past, population aging was a problem mainly in developed countries, but today it is gaining importance in developing countries (DCs), going from a marginal issue to a major concern whose effects are felt in all aspects of life. According to United Nations statistics, the number of elderly people will increase from 600 million in 2000 to 2 billion in 2050. They will represent 6% of the population of developing countries (Madrid Action Plan on Ageing, 2002). In Cameroon, with 19.4 million inhabitants, the elderly (60 years and older) represent 5.5% of the country's population (3rd RGPH) and more than half (55%) are women. [11]

The WHO notes that until the initiatives taken in the last quarter of the 20th century to combat domestic violence and child abuse, elder abuse was a phenomenon confined to the private domain and carefully hidden from the public. Today, it is increasingly seen as a significant problem that is likely to grow, given the rapid aging of the population in many countries. [12]

Note that the problem of elder abuse exists in both developing and developed countries, although it is generally underestimated worldwide. Prevalence rates or estimates exist only in some developed countries - they range from 1 to 10%. Although the extent of elder abuse is unknown, its social and moral importance is clear. As such, it calls for a multi-faceted global response that focuses on protecting the rights of older persons. Approaches to defining, detecting and responding to elder abuse must be placed in a cultural context and considered alongside culture-specific risk factors. [13]

The consequences of abuse can be particularly severe in the elderly, as their bones are more fragile and recovery time is longer. Even a relatively minor injury can have serious and permanent consequences. As with other types of abuse, elder abuse includes physical, sexual and psychological abuse, as well as neglect. Older adults are particularly vulnerable to the risk of extortion, that is, misuse of their money and resources by relatives or caregivers. [14]

In the WHO report cited above, it is noted that there appear to be certain situations that put older adults at particular risk of violence. In some cases, already strained relationships within the family may worsen as a result of stress and frustration as the older person loses independence. In others, the conflict may be due to the caregiver's dependence on the older person for housing or financial reasons. Social isolation is also a major risk factor. Many older people are left out of the

---

[11] Marcel NKOMA, *La sécurité sociale des personnes âgées en question*, Workshop with the Ministry of Economy, Planning and Land Management, Cameroon, 2011, available at http://www.ceped.org/cdrom/meknes/spipcddf.htmParticle33, accessed May 17, 2014 at 1:30 p.m.
[12] WHO Report , *Elder Abuse*, 2012, P1, available at http://www.who.int/violenceinjury prevention, accessed March 24, 2014 at 11:15 am.
[13] WHO report, *Ageing and the life course*, 2012 available at http://www.who.int/ageing/projects/elderabuse/en/,accessed March 24, 2014 at 11:15 am.
[14] WHO report, *Elder Abuse*, 2012, op cit.

loop because of physical or mental disabilities or are left alone because of the loss of friends and family members. [15]

Worldwide, nearly 36 million people are affected by Alzheimer's disease. Alzheimer's disease is a phenomenon that has grown over the last 20 years. There will be more than 22 million people over the age of 60 by 2050. According to statistics, here's what's in store for this disease in the future: The number of Alzheimer's patients is expected to double in 20 years worldwide, reaching 65.7 million cases by 2035. According to the association of third age people of France, the number of people affected by Alzheimer's disease in 2050 should be 2 million according to estimates. According to INSEE, one person out of 4 over 65 years old could be affected by Alzheimer's disease by 2020, that is to say 1.3 million French people. [16]

In Africa, the majority of the third age people work in the informal sector in spite of their advanced age, they continue to work and to support their families until the moment of their extinction [17] from that, it is necessary to point out that not only the third age people constitute the group of the invalids but also they constitute a category of the active population following the conjuncture of the world life [18]

Speaking of the situation of the elderly in Africa, the WHO in Ghana shows that Ghanaians are living longer. The proportion of the population over 60 years of age is expected to reach 12% by 2050, up from 7% in 2010. The Ministry of Health is working with WHO and its partners to help older Ghanaians live healthier and more productive lives. In 2010, the Ghanaian government approved a national policy on aging. Two years later, it asked WHO to help it move from theory to practice through the establishment of nursing homes. In Ghana, more than 4,000 people aged 50 and over were interviewed as part of the SAGE study. They provided information on their household, economic and social status, health behavior, diagnosis and treatment of chronic diseases, and access to health services. Their weight and height were recorded as well as blood pressure and lung capacity. After this analysis, a decision was taken by the Ghanaian government in partnership with WHO to set up a system to protect the elderly by establishing homes or nursing homes for them. [19]

In DRC, the situation of the old people's homes is justified by the fact that the Director of the old people's home of KABINDA, in the commune of LINGWALA in Kinshasa, expressed on Wednesday, the wish for the Congolese State to adopt a law on the protection of the elderly in the Democratic Republic of Congo, as one of the lasting solutions to the acts of indignation of which

---

[15] Id.
[16] WHO report, *Elder Abuse*, 2012, op cit.
[17] HEAL PAGE Report: *Africa's Ageing Problem:* Summary, (unpublished), Nairobi, 2000
[18] MUMBERE MUHASA Charmant, *problematic of the socio-economic situation of the elderly in the city of Goma*, Dissertation (unpublished), ISDR GL, 2012, P4.
[19] WHO, *Ghana Takes Care of its Aging Population*, October 2013 available at http://www.who.int/features/2013/ghana-living-longer/fr/, accessed March 24, 2014 at 10:30 a.m.

these people are victims. [20]

According to Mrs. Molopo who spoke to the ACP, the Home for the Elderly of Kabinda registers every week cases of family rejection of this social category on behalf of close relatives, who generally put forward unfounded reasons including the presumption of witchcraft. She maintained that the vote of this law will allow the DRC to obtain an instrument of size for the judicial pursuit of all those who would worry this vulnerable section of the Congolese, adding that in the meantime provisions should be taken by the police in view of the protection and the daily security of the elderly throughout the country. [21]

Speaking about the functioning of this Home for the Elderly, Mrs. Molopo revealed that it is in an unviable situation due to the lack of premises, beds and mosquito nets, taking into account the importance of the ever-increasing demand, in addition to the permanent need for assistance in food, detergents and other non-food items. The Kabinda Home takes care of about 31 inpatient units compared to 75 outpatient units in the commune of Lingwala alone. According to her, the government should provide an annual budget for the care of these people, without forgetting their access to health care as well as to various recreational and entertainment activities. [22]

In Kisangani, five residents of the old people's home in Tshopo have died in recent months as a result of poor nutrition and precarious housing conditions. Those in charge of this site are sounding the alarm to the local authorities. [23]

The life in the home of the old people in Kinshasa, a second childhood, these last ones claim by saying. To manage the elderly, seems to be a real apostolate for the staff of the old people's home. To house and feed the elderly, here is the work that some people initiated in the maintenance of old people give themselves, on a daily basis. The old people's home of the commune of Kintambo is the perfect illustration of this job whose main mission is to manage the gerontological whims. [24]

Similarly, the Democratic Republic of Congo (DRC) has (approximately) 3.5% of elderly people. These people are not all vulnerable, but neither do they live in decent (normal) conditions due to the precarious state of the majority of the population and the resignation of the State in the socio-economic and cultural fields. The elderly, who are supposed to benefit from family support, suffer the same fate as their protectors, i.e. 78.5% of the population (total) living under the weight of misery. Several causes are at the root of the vulnerability of the elderly. These are the galloping deterioration of the socio-economic situation leading to the increasing impoverishment of the population, the

---

[20] Ms. Molopo, *Nécessité d'une loi de protection des personnes de troisième âge en RDC*, 2012 available at http://www.acpcongo.com/index.php?option=com content&view=article&id=27837:rd-congo. Accessed May 17, 2014.
[21] Ms. Molopo, *Nécessité d'une loi de protection des personnes de troisième âge en RDC*, op cit.
[22] Id.
[23] Marcel NGOMBO, Interview with the Provincial Minister in charge of Public Health, Social Affairs, Solidarity and Family on the precarious living conditions at the TSHOPO home for the elderly, available at http://radiookapi.net/regions/province-orientale/2013/10/03/province-orientale-conditions-de-vie-precaire-au- home-des-vieillards-de-la-tshopo/#.U3fEOT upK4, accessed on May 17, 2014 at 1:30 pm.
[24] http://www.laprosperiteonline.net/show.php?id=13825&rubrique=Nation

displacement of the population and the urban demographic explosion, the disappearance of traditional family models, the inadequacy of basic social services, particularly hospitals and geriatrics, and retrograde customs. [25]

With regard to retrograde customs in particular, many tribes do not tolerate, for example, the presence of a son-in-law next to his mother-in-law, nor of a daughter-in-law next to her father-in-law. In urban areas, because of the promiscuity that characterizes Congolese households (60% occupy a two-bedroom house), the elderly

is too much in a family. A grandfather or grandmother, for example, cannot share the same room with his or her grandchildren. Many customs weaken the elderly to the point of abandonment. On the other hand, children who agree to live with their elderly parents often lack the means to support them. The vulnerability of the elderly can be seen in their health, food and housing: the disengagement of the State in the health sector does not allow them to benefit from proper medical care; dieticians do not take charge of their diet; these elderly people live in abandoned buildings, markets and railway stations where they live without basic hygiene conditions for the rest of their lives. Very few elderly people are taken in by the hospices where they find a new life. The so-called "wizards" are automatically declared non grata and driven out of the house because they represent a danger of death.
[26]

Apart from the problem related to custom, all the other causes of the vulnerability of the elderly revolve around a common point, namely poverty. As a consequence, the vulnerability of the elderly leads to their marginalization from society and family, exploitation by the economic and social environment, de-socialization, exposure to disease, stress due to lack of affection, shortening of their life span and abandonment. In rural areas, the elderly are generally highly respected; they are a living library, even a reference for young people. [27]

In the province of North Kivu, the management of elderly people (age > 60 years) living in Butembo/North Kivu Province/East of the DR Congo is a crucial problem and more relevant than the management of diabetes mellitus.

In Butembo and its surroundings, the elderly (age > 60) lack appropriate multi-support: psychological, medical, nutritional and hygienic; and yet, these people have the right to human dignity, for having made us what we are today. [28]

Most of these people are economically deprived and disabled, and no longer have any professional activity that could generate financial income; their income is nil, which makes it financially impossible to control and monitor their health. [29]

Physiologically weakened, these people present an associated poly pathology (diabetes, arterial hypertension, acute respiratory infections, rheumatism, anemia, cataract, blindness, nephritis, polyneuritis, parasitosis, dermatosis, multi-facial malnutrition, stress, depression, anxiety, ...). This poly pathology, not monitored or poorly taken care of in Butembo, leads to many handicaps; and a

---

[25] LA voix des sans - voix (VSV), *Rapport d'information sur les personnes âgées à Kinshasa/R.D.C*, July 1999, available at http://www.congonline.com/vsv/rapports/rapports1/07.htm.

[26] LA VOIX DES SANS - VOIX (VSV), *Rapport d'information sur les personnes âgées à Kinshasa/R.D.C*, July 1999, op cit.
[27] Id.
[28] George MUSAVULI, care for the elderly, assistance program, BUTEMBO, August 2011, available on http://www.congoforum.be/fr/nieuwsdetail.asp?subitem=3&newsid=179865&Actualiteit=selected, accessed on March 24, 2014 at 10:30 AM.
[29] Same as

large number of elderly people are thus prematurely disabled. [30]

Socially abandoned to themselves, these people suffer from a multiple lack: psychological, medical, nutritional and hygienic; which explains their poor health marked by a poly pathological chronicity. In Goma and its surroundings in Eastern DR Congo, no preparation as a home for the elderly seems to be in place to meet the needs of appropriate care (psychological, medical, nutritional and hygienic) that this situation of gerontology suggests: this is so from the point of view of infrastructure, personnel, equipment as well as therapeutic strategies and knowledge. [31]

As the city of Goma in general and in particular the health zone of Goma is not spared by the problems of supervision of the old people speaking about the conditions of life and which slaughters a total number of 19586 people of the third ages (55 to 85 years and more). The city of Goma, does not have any retirement home or home for the elderly while they are faced with multiple difficult situations such as abuse within their families, stress and frustration that leads to trauma, physical disabilities, the state of vulnerability for some and the persistence of diseases that can lead them to situations of death. [32]

In the city of Goma, the elderly live in despicable conditions, they are not supervised by any private or state organization, this leads to a spirit of begging on their part in all the alleys of the city, we have made certain observations that every Friday and Wednesday, the elderly are grouped in clusters along the stores and stores of individuals to find something to eat, this state of affairs shows without relaunching that there is a problem of supervision of these people who made us
Growing up with their sons, today the weight of age has made them vulnerable, miserable on the socio-economic level but strong in spirit and experience.

Note that in 2013, the commune of Goma, where the Goma health zone is located, experienced a number of deaths, including deaths among the elderly. The number of cases of deaths for the third age people was 12 cases of which 8 men and 4 women. During the last month of the year only (December 2012), 4 cases were registered, of which 3 were men and one was a woman, all of them old people. But let's note that for the year 2012 the crude mortality rate for old people was 11%. This is due to the lack of appropriate psychological, medical, nutritional and hygienic support that is not done by the health zone of Goma, but also the inappropriate living conditions (poor) of these people due to a poverty of the population especially within their families. [33]

As far as diseases are concerned, people of the third age present associated pathologies such as. diabetes, arterial hypertension, acute respiratory infections, rheumatism, anaemia, cataract,

---

[30] Id.
[31] Id.
[32] Bureau de l'état civil, commune de Goma, census report by age group, 2013.
[33] Pre-survey with the nurse supervisor of the Goma health zone on March 30, 2014 at 8:30 am.

blindness, nephritis, polyneuritis, parasitosis, dermatosis, multi-facial malnutrition, stress, depression, anguish, ...) When these pathologies are not supervised or are badly taken care of, they cause a lot of handicaps; and a great number of people of the third age are thus precociously invalid and precipitate death. It should be noted that the health zone of Goma has no future prospects for the elderly, due to the lack of funding to address this project. [34]

1.3. Research Questions
1.3.1. General question

This study is based on an overarching and master question formulated as follows:

What are the needs for the establishment of homes for the elderly experienced by the elderly in the health zone of Goma?

1.3.2. Specific questions

The following specific questions have emerged from this research, including

> What are the housing conditions for the elderly in the Goma health zone?
> What are the housing needs of the elderly in the Goma health zone?
> What are the types of housing orientations expressed by the elderly in the Goma health zone?

1.4. Research Hypotheses

A hypothesis is an anticipated answer to the question that the researcher asks himself at the beginning of his project or research. In view of the theme presented above, we believe that :

> Food insecurity, psycho-physical mistreatment, disrepute within their families, low financial contribution would be conditions of accommodation of the elderly in the health zone of Goma;
> The premises adapted to their physical conditions, the desire to live in the home, the need to protect their integuments would be housing needs experienced by the elderly in the health zone of Goma;
> Social assistance, family aid, psychological support, medical care, economic assistance through IGAs would be the types of orientations expressed by the elderly in the health zone of Goma.

1.5. Objectives of the research
1.5.1. General objective

The overall objective of this study is to

Assess the needs for the establishment of homes for the elderly experienced by the elderly in the health zone of Goma.

1.5.2. Specific Objectives:

Specifically, the following objectives are formulated:

> To evaluate the housing conditions of the elderly in the health zone of Goma;
> To assess the housing needs of the elderly in the health zone of Goma;

---
[34] Id.

> Determine the types of housing orientations expressed by the ᵉˡᵈᵉʳˡʸ ⁱⁿ ᵗʰᵉ Goma health zone.

1.6. Choice and interest of the subject

The choice of this subject is justified by the scientific interest that we have in the health field, particularly the health of the third age (elderly).

However, the choice is justified by the fact that the population of the health zone of Goma in general and more specifically the third age people are not in their turn spared by the problem of management and living conditions because the major part of this old population cover a population in which situations of abuse, The stress and frustration that leads to trauma, physical disabilities, vulnerability, illnesses due to the lack of support by the services of care for these vulnerable people.

In fact, the rejection of the practices of care for the elderly within their respective families, even outside the family, the non-application of psychological techniques to better live with these people, the social and cultural conceptions of the population in front of the elderly, lead us to a major concern that gnaws at all nations, especially us, who want to carry out this study in order to see how the elderly can live in appropriate conditions and extend their life expectancy. On the other hand, this work will be a scientific reference for other researchers who will orient their studies in this field.

1.7. Spatio - temporal delimitation a. In time

This study (investigation) being over a period of time from January 2014 through July 2014.

b. In space

This study is entitled "*Study on the needs for the establishment of homes for the elderly experienced by the ᵉˡᵈᵉʳˡʸ in the health area of Goma*. We are going to carry out this study in the health zone of Goma located in the commune of Goma, city of GOMA in the province of North Kivu and indeed in DRC.

1.8. Definition of key concepts

- **Study:** Methodical application of the mind seeking to learn and understand. It is an effort to acquire knowledge, an ordered series of work and exercises necessary for instruction. [35]
- **Need:** Natural necessity, lack of a necessary thing that one desires. [36]
- **Home :** Home for the reception and accommodation of people[37].
- **Old man:** Man or woman of a great age. [38]
- **Health zone: This is** the peripheral, operational unit of the national health system, the basic unit of health planning at two levels (network of health centers and a general reference hospital). [39]

---

[35] Dictionary, le robert de poche, paris, 2009. P269.
[36] Id.
[37] Same as
[38] Dictionary, le robert de poche, paris, 2009, op cit.
[39] Ministry of Health, 2002.

- **Health: it is** a state of physical, mental and social well-being, not only consisting in the absence of disease or infirmity. [40]

---

[40] Prof. Dr. KAMBALE KARAFULI Léopold, *public health course*, (unpublished), ULPGL/GOMA, G1FSDC, 2013 2014, P6.

Chapter Two.
REVIEW OF THE LITERATURE

11.1. Introduction

This chapter, which concerns the review of the research literature, aims to collect information from other researchers who have dealt with themes similar to the needs for the establishment of homes for the elderly experienced by the ^{third} age people. As if to say that it is a question of being inspired by the previous studies carried out by other researchers around the needs of the establishment of homes and/or old people's homes in favor of the old people (third age people). At the end of this chapter, we present a summary of this literature review through the schematization of the conceptual and operational framework. The questions and hypotheses dictate the subpoints of this chapter. In addition to the introduction, general information on homes for the elderly, the summary of the literature review and the research framework, this chapter has three main sub-sections:

> Housing conditions for the ^{elderly};
> Housing needs experienced by ^{seniors};
> Types of housing referrals expressed by seniors.

11.2. General information on the elderly

According to the gerontologist doctor Pierre GUILLET, quoted by MUMBERE MUHASA Charmant, "aging well" is based on the balance of five pillars: finances, health, social life, intellectual life must be available in the life of an elderly person, the American criteria of a good aging are:

- A life span longer than the national life expectancy;
- Good health: one or more diseases treated and blocked in their evolution;
- A feeling of well-being

The old people must finish their existences without material concern, growing old is a natural process that concerns all of us, this process should be followed by a good reception otherwise, we should know that women and men ages are useful for our societies. The dysfunction linked to the process of aging, if they are avoidable they contribute largely to take the people of ^{3rd} age vulnerable, their impact depends however on the individuals, of their environment, this dysfunction can be noticed on the economic, social and sanitary plan. [41]

On the economic level: the persistent crisis has increased the poverty and the difficulties of the living conditions of the ^{third} age people who live in a certain extreme precariousness causing the non-satisfaction of the primary needs as the food and the housing, it is estimated to 8,2% of the ^{third} age people who benefit from a security of a housing of which they are themselves owners, whereas 91,8%

---

[41] MUMBERE MUHASA Charmant, *problématique de la situation socioéconomique des personnes de troisième âge dans la ville de Goma*, Mémoire (inédit), ISDR GL, 2012, p5-6.

are without fixed housing, on the social level, the ᵗʰⁱʳᵈ age people suffer from the problem of the integration and the acceptance in the society, what makes that they are taxed of all the evils as: the contempt, the rejection, the witchcraft, this last fact that one declares it they are worth nothing they undergo pursuits to such points that they are driven out in the houses because, it is considered as source of the death, on the socio-cultural plan, the consequences of the changes on the situation of the old people are multiple. Those who were once considered the guardians of the community and ancestral values, are not protected by their families or by their community. In terms of health, the elderly are affected by diseases and chronic pathologies such as hypertension, diabetes, rheumatism, cancer and others. [42]

As Mohammed Bedruni points out in his article on the characteristics and conditions of social and health care for Moroccan and Algerian elderly people - similarities and dissimilarities - nowadays, the importance of population ageing as a major social fact is practically unanimous. For a long time, the latter was considered a phenomenon specific to Western societies, which led to the reduction of its social and geographical scope. Unfortunately, this view has been contradicted by the facts. The increasingly available demographic statistics confirm that aging is rather a global phenomenon linked to the demographic transition. Its magnitude will inevitably disrupt Western societies but also and especially those of developing countries. Projections by the United Nations Population Division predict that the number of people aged 60 and over will triple by 2050. This will increase the number of people aged 60 and over from about 630 million today to nearly 2 billion. The majority of these people (80%) will live in developing countries, knowing that their aging process will develop at a faster pace than in developed countries. Thus, if for France it took more than 127 years to reduce its percentage of elderly people (60 years and older) from 10 to 20%, China would need barely 27 years to make the same transition. It should also be noted that while rich, industrialized countries consider the problem of aging to be a real challenge, both for

---

[42] MUMBERE MUHASA Charmant, *problématique de la situation socioéconomique des personnes de troisième âge dans la ville de Goma*, op cit.

For their present and their future, developing countries would have to face the same challenge with more acuity and fewer resources, as G.H. Brundtland, director of the WHO, put it: "Developed countries became rich before they became old, developing countries will be old before they become rich". Aware of the large number and the heterogeneity that characterizes the countries in this last category, we had to restrict the field of exploration for the preparation of this contribution to two countries in the Maghreb and North African geographical area. [43]

11.3. Accommodation conditions for the elderly

11.3.1. Food insecurity

The way we eat is very important for the elderly, because the quality of our diet helps to slow down the natural aging process, delay the onset of certain age-related diseases, and therefore to age with a good quality of life.

According to Béatrice CARRAZ, from a nutritional point of view, the major risk in the elderly is a risk linked to malnutrition and deficiencies, and not really to overload: the important points to check remain the energy intake, the intake of proteins, calcium and essential fatty acids. Protein-energy malnutrition favors the onset of dependence by weakening the body's natural defenses. For this author, the needs of the elderly are identical to those of adults, no more and no less. However, food consumption decreases: less meat, fewer real meals, severe dietary restrictions due to health problems (cholesterol, salt, sugar...). And this type of behavior plays on the quality of life and the evolution towards dependencies. [44]

The social elders of Adjamé-village, according to their culture, eat mainly attiéké (Agbodjama) made with cassava, but also foutou or foufou (cocotcha) of yam or plantain. These dishes are accompanied by "claire" sauce, "graine" sauce or "N'tro" sauce with "good" fish specific to the lagoon such as broché, machoiron, captain, fished directly in the lagoon. However, with the current pollution of the lagoon, fishing is no longer practiced by the villagers. [45]

11.3.2. Psychophysical abuse

According to the WHO, between 1995 and 2025, the number of people over 60 years of age worldwide is expected to at least double, from 542 million to some 1.2 billion, of a care facility reported witnessing physical abuse of an elderly patient at least once in the past year, 10% admitted to at least one act of physical abuse themselves, and 40% reported psychologically harassing patients. Institutional abuse also includes the use of physical restraint against the elderly, disrespect for patients' dignity and freedom of choice in daily life, or lack of care (e.g., resulting in pressure sores).

---

[43] Mohammed BEDROUNI, *Characteristics and conditions of social and health care of the Moroccan and Algerian elderly Ressemblances et dissemblances*, in la vieillesse au sud approche comparative, Art, university of saad Daheleb of blida, Algeria, March 2011.
[44] BéatriceCARRAZ, *L'alimentation des personnes âgées*, Paris 2001, p11.
[45] Ahou Clémentine TANOH, *Etude sur les conditions de vie des personnes âgées en côte d'Ivoire*: Regard sur la maltraitance à Adjame Village, université de COCODY, (unpublished), Thèse, Abidjan 2006-2007.

According to Ahou Clémentine TANOH cited above, elder abuse has remained until recently, a phenomenon unknown, denied, not subject to any study or, a fortiori, prevention. Elderly abuse is still quite secret and is developing both in families and in institutions. In the family, research has shown that violence is a habitual way of life in 20% of families, violence against all the weak members of the family: children, women and the elderly. Also, several studies have shown that adolescents who abuse their parents have often been abused children themselves. When they become adults, the silent abused children, in front of the power of their parents, reveal themselves in their turn abusers, when with the advance in age, their parents weaken physically and intellectually. [47]

For Hugonot (2003), quoted by Ahou Clémentine TANOH, it shows that it is by the exhaustion of tolerance that one arrives at violence towards the elderly. In the relationship with the elderly, it can happen that the behavior of one of the two partners reaches such a repetitive or excessive level that it exhausts the tolerance of the other. This can lead to statements such as "*I couldn't take it anymore, she wore me down, so I slapped her.* "It is therefore the tolerance that breaks down and the idea of rejection that is born. In the old couple, continues the author, the violence is most often related to a reversal of power. Because of intellectual decline and increased age, the dominant spouse is now dependent on the previously dominated spouse, who often becomes the primary caregiver. Domestic violence against the elderly is often related to the character traits, attitudes and behaviors of the elderly. According to Hugonot, we find in the literature many portraits of obnoxious, tyrannical and defiant old men. Withdrawn on their "money", such as Arpagon, or naturally hostile to their family or social environment on which they reject their refusal to grow old, to live a life henceforth too long and alone, unable to mourn their youth or to assume their widowhood. [48]

Elderly people are abused both in the family and in institutions. In both cases, there are several categories of abuse. The most frequent forms of abuse are financial and psychological (27% each). In the financial area, it is not only the withholding of pensions, thefts, swindles, anticipated inheritance, robbery of money, movable and immovable goods, but also living off the grandparents. Physical abuse (15% of the reported cases) includes beatings, slaps, and untreated or badly treated bedsores. Less known than the previous ones, but very numerous (15%) are the neglects of daily life assistance, voluntary or not: getting up, going to bed, washing, eating, walking. To these must be added murder, deliberate assault and battery, rape, tying to a bed or chair, inadequate feeding, etc.

---

[46] WHO, *Elder Abuse* Report, August 2011, available at http://www.who.int/mediacentre/factsheets/fs357/fr/.
[47] Ahou Clémentine TANOH, *Etude sur les conditions de vie des personnes âgées en côte d'Ivoire*: Regard sur la maltraitance à Adjame Village, op cit.
[48] Ahou Clémentine TANOH, *Etude sur les conditions de vie des personnes âgées en côte d'Ivoire*: Regard sur la maltraitance à Adjame Village, op cit.

Medication abuse (4-5% of reported cases) which is the excess of medication, neuroleptics or, conversely, deprivation of medication and care. In addition, it is necessary to note the violation of the rights of the elderly and their active neglect (authoritarian placement, confinement...) and passive neglect (forgetfulness, self neglect).

According to Robert Hugonot and Françoise Busby quoted by Ahou Clémentine TANOH, the majority of victims are widowed women (75%) living in families. Men (25%) are mistreated by their spouses, a family member or by a third person, a companion of "some time", an abusive companion. [49]

11.3.3. Disregard within families

Valérie GOLAZ and Philippe ANTOINE in an article on the living conditions and vulnerability of the elderly in the South, a comparative study between Uganda and Senegal, state that the vast majority of elderly people live with other adults, elderly or not. Men, in particular, are more likely than women to live with other adults, largely due to the earlier widowhood of women. In Senegal, almost the entire older population is in this situation. In Uganda, compared to other African countries, there is a large proportion of elderly people living alone (more than 12% compared to 1% in Senegal). In Uganda, this situation is more frequent for men living in urban areas (15%). It is less common for elderly women who also live in urban areas, which may be attributed to the fact that the majority of men migrate to the city to work. The result in Uganda is a significant nuclearization of households. Living alone does not necessarily mean being far from any relatives, as most isolated elderly people live in close proximity to other related households. However, like Zimmer and Dayton (2005), co-residence can be seen as providing greater physical and emotional support than mere spatial proximity without co-residence. Ugandan women, both rural and urban, are more likely than men to be single with children under 15 years of age (8-10% of women and only 2% of men). About half of these cases involve one child, but the other half involve several. In Uganda, the older the person, the more likely he or she is to live alone, especially for women. This situation is very marginal in Senegal and there is little change in the situation according to age. [50]

11.3.4. Low financial contribution

Maryse GAIMARD and Benoit LIBALI, for the DRC, say that unlike in developed countries, the majority of the elderly population in the Congo is still active. More than half (52%) report being employed (49% of men and 54% of women). Retired persons, or those who have declared themselves as such, represent 17 percent of the population aged 60 or more; this proportion rises to 36 percent among the male population. Women who do not declare a professional activity say they are

---

[49] Id.
[50] Valérie GOLAZ and Philippe ANTOINE, *Living conditions and vulnerability of the elderly in the South:* What are the elderly in a vulnerable situation, comparative study between Uganda and Senegal, art, France, March 2011.

housewives (29%) and more rarely retired (3%). These proportions vary little with age, contrary to what one might think. The proportion of older men with a job is around 50% between the ages of 60 and 69, and then remains at around 45%; the proportion of retirees decreases from the age of 80 onwards (falling below 30%) in favor of an "other" category. In the female population, the proportion of women declaring to be active, from 58 to 60 % between 60 and 69 years of age, falls to around 50 % between 70 and 79 years of age and then decreases to a quarter of the population. The decline in these proportions is also to the benefit of the "other" category and that of housewives. In total, the elderly population is still very often active and more than 90% of them declare their professional status as self-employed. This situation reflects a high level of precariousness in the economic activities of the Congolese, dominated by the informal sector; until around the year 2000, only 5% of the Congolese working population carried out an economic activity in the modern formal sector. [51]

11.4. Housing needs experienced by seniors

In a study conducted by Ahou Clémentine TANOH on Living conditions of the elderly in Côte d'Ivoire: A look at the abuse in Adjame Village, the results showed that the vast majority of the elderly - 86% of those over 75 years old - live in ordinary housing. Moreover, more than 50% of women over 75 and nearly a quarter of men of the same age live alone. It is true that in the 1990's, many homes for the elderly were repaired, properly equipped and adapted. However, the lack of elevators in many buildings is a serious problem. Seniors also face daily difficulties in housing that is narrow for those who use wheelchairs and other aids in their movements. In addition, one in four seniors feel that stores, the post office, bank, pharmacy and/or health services are located too far from their homes. Also in the 1990s, living in a housing and service center became more common than any other form of senior services, replacing institutional care. [52]

11.4.1. Premises adapted to physical conditions

According to Ahou Clémentine TANOH quoted above, her study stipulates that most of the houses belong to the indigenous families of this city. Thus, all the elderly people interviewed in this study declare that they own their homes. The men are entirely owners. The women, on the other hand, are either living with their husbands, in their husbands' families, or in their own families, depending on their present and, above all, past marital status. In total, regardless of gender, none of the elderly interviewed rent the house in which they live. However, these homeowners complain about the cramped conditions of their homes as a result of urbanization. The yards are crowded. And it is to remedy the problem of promiscuity that those who have the means, build in height. In addition, the noise coming from vehicles, shops, passers-by and schools makes it impossible for these elderly

---

[51] Maryse GAIMARD and Benoit LIBALI, *Vieillissement et conditions de vie des personnes âgées en République du Congo*, Art, Op cit.
[52] Ahou Clémentine TANOH, *Etude sur les conditions de vie des personnes âgées en côte d'Ivoire*: Regard sur la maltraitance à Adjame Village, op cit.

people to rest. It is the place to mention the environmental pollution and the inopportune visits of the bandits. [53]

Esther Chrystelle EYINGA DIMI says that access to decent housing for the elderly is also a social protection issue for this category of the population. The elderly also encounter many difficulties due to the inadequacy of their residential environment with the requirements of their health condition. This situation is all the more disadvantageous for elderly people in the countryside or in poorly built areas where housing may lack comfort and access may be difficult. This section focuses on their access to decent housing, clean water and electricity. Older people who own their own homes can, to some extent, be considered as having housing security: 91.8% of older people live in homes that they own, while 8.2% of them face housing insecurity. However, when we look at their housing status, we see that 29.1% of them live in low-standard housing and 43.1% in traditional housing (improved or simple). A small proportion, 6.2%, live in precarious housing. We also note that 45.3% of the elderly do not have access to clean water. [54]

Similarly, 67.6% of elderly households do not have access to electricity. Although more than two-thirds of these households have access to electricity in urban areas, a significant proportion still use kerosene (28.5%) and wood/coal (3.1%) in urban areas. In rural areas, on the other hand, kerosene lighting is the preferred method: 69.8% of elderly households use it. Given that the price of a liter of oil has risen sharply in recent years, one might deduce that the expense of buying oil, which is in fact an incompressible need, could further strain the already hypothetical income of the elderly. Finally, 84.4% of the elderly use wood or charcoal to cook their food, 72.4% in urban areas and 90.5% in rural areas. [55]

According to Maryse GAIMARD and Benoit LIBALI, cited above, the homes of the elderly are made of cinder blocks (26%), fired bricks (19%), unfired bricks (19%), planks (12%), or clay (15%). The lower proportion of solid houses among the elderly compared to the total (34%) is explained by the greater rurality of the elderly. In fact, cinder block is mainly used in cities, whereas in the countryside the dominant material is rammed earth (30% of rural households), followed by fired or unfired brick

(20 %). There are no significant differences according to the gender of the head of the household or according to age. More than three-quarters of the roofs are made of durable materials (sheet metal, tile or concrete), compared to 82% for all households, and nearly 20% of the roofs are made of straw; the latter is most common in rural areas, where it covers nearly half of the houses. Only 46% of homes

---

[53] Ahou Clémentine TANOH, *Etude sur les conditions de vie des personnes âgées en côte d'Ivoire*: Regard sur la maltraitance à Adjame Village, op cit.
[54] Esther Chrystelle EYINGA DIMI, *Living conditions and vulnerability of the elderly in the South*, Socioeconomic situations of the elderly in Cameroon, Art, Université Bordeaux Segalen, Centre Émile Durkheim - CEPED, March 2011.
[55] Id.

have hard floors (cement or tiles), compared with 63% of all households; more than half (52%) of households headed by elderly persons still have a dirt floor (33% of all households). Dirt floors are found mainly in the countryside (82% of houses) and in semi-urban areas (60%). In the city, more than 80% of homes have cement floors. The floor is more often hard when the head of the household is a man (50%) and dirt when the head is a woman (58%). In total, dwellings headed by people aged 60 or older are less frequently made of durable materials than for all households. The difference is due to the greater rurality of older households. Dwellings headed by women aged 60 or older are smaller on average than those headed by older men. For example, 44% of elderly female-headed households have only one bedroom in their dwelling, compared to 21% of men. However, elderly people living alone in their dwelling represent only 21% of household heads. [56]

Conversely, when the head of household is male, dwellings are more likely to have three bedrooms (23% vs. 15%) or four bedrooms (30% vs. 12%). Dwellings are on average larger in rural areas, especially for all households. Access to electricity is also less common among older households: 23% versus 35% for all households. The type of energy used by the elderly is most often oil (73%), followed by electricity (22%). Other energy sources are negligible (2.5% use wood for lighting). There are very slight gender differences: men use electricity slightly more often (25%) than women (20%), with the balance shifting to oil. These households, which are headed by elderly people, appear to be less well equipped than households as a whole, with electricity less often available (33 percent of all households use electricity and 60 percent use oil). However, in rural and semi-urban areas, 88% and 81% of households use oil, while in urban areas 51% of households use electricity. [57]

For cooking, the most used energy source is firewood (64% vs. 41% in all households) followed by coal (18%). Gas is used for cooking by only 9% of the elderly and oil by 7%. Electricity is hardly used for cooking (2%). Women use wood a little more than men, but the difference is small (65% vs. 60% of men) and slightly less coal, oil, but especially gas. Wood is the overall energy source in rural (88% of households) and semi-urban areas (69%); in urban areas it is used by only 14% of households, compared to 41% for charcoal. [58]

More than 80% of elderly households have access to a source of drinking water: 22% of the elderly have a tap in the plot, 17% have a tap outside the plot, 18% have a well or borehole, and 26% have a spring. There are no disparities in the source of drinking water by gender of the heads of household or between elderly households and all households. [59]

---

[56] Maryse GAIMARD and Benoit LIBALI, *Vieillissement et conditions de vie des personnes âgées en République du Congo*, Art, Université Bordeaux Segalen, Centre Émile Durkheim - CEPED, France March 2011.
[57] Maryse GAIMARD and Benoit LIBALI, *Vieillissement et conditions de vie des personnes âgées en République du Congo*, Art, Université Bordeaux Segalen, Centre Émile Durkheim - CEPED, France March 2011.
[58] Id.
[59] Id.

Sanitation facilities are still traditional for most seniors. This is the case for the shower: more than half (52%) of those aged 60 or more have a traditional shower and almost a quarter (22%) go to the stream to wash themselves. The semi-modern shower is used by only 11% of the elderly and the modern shower by 9% of them (4% in the dwelling and 5% in the plot). Again, there are no significant differences by gender. The differences are also small with the general population (53% use the traditional shower and 13% the modern shower). On the other hand, the place of residence is a more determining factor of comfort. In urban areas, nearly 20% of Congolese have a modern shower and 20% have a semi-modern shower. In semi-urban areas, 70% use the traditional shower, and in rural areas, nearly 50% (47%) use the water course and 37% the traditional shower. [60]

Nearly 20% of elderly households do not have a toilet in their home. The most common type of toilet facility is a latrine in the plot (63%). In addition, 16% of the elderly do not have a toilet and relieve themselves in the open. 12% have a modern toilet (4% in the dwelling and 8% in the plot) and 8% have a pit that can be emptied, slightly more often among the male population. Here again, the elderly are less well equipped than the population as a whole, no doubt in connection with their more rural habitat, which is less often equipped with a modern toilet and where latrines in the plot and recourse to nature (33%) are still very common. [61]

The sewage disposal system is also very rudimentary. Nearly 60% (57%) of the elderly have their water drained in the plot and 22% in the street. Only 5% of the elderly use a cesspool or a gutter. The level of equipment is always slightly lower for women than for all households, where a greater proportion is evacuated into the street. One quarter of elderly households have a garbage collection system: 14% of the elderly give their garbage to a private collection system and 10% throw it in a public garbage can. In 49% of the cases it is left on the plot and in 15% it is thrown away in the street. Differences are more pronounced between living environments than between older and non-elderly households. [62]

11.4.2. The wish to live in the home

In a comparative study on the perception of the care of elderly Lebanese, Moroccan and Senegalese, conducted by Nicole CAMPUIS LUCCIANI et al, the results state that more than 20% of Senegalese living in Senegal, a country where there are no retirement homes, say they would accept living in a specialized institution. They would be able to rest; they would feel safer; they would be cared for; their families would be relieved; they would be reunited with people of their own age; they would like regular visits from their families. The majority of the Senegalese responses were negative, however, because they relied mainly on their children; it would be an abandonment, it is not a place

---
[60] Id.
[61] Maryse GAIMARD and Benoit LIBALI, *Vieillissement et conditions de vie des personnes âgées en République du Congo*, op cit.
[62] Id.

of fulfillment; it is not in their culture; they do not intend to stay in France if they have to "go through this". All the Moroccans in France refused the idea of a retirement home, mentioning the family that could help them, a return to their family in Morocco, unless they were forced to do so by illness. The Lebanese are mostly against it, evoking shame, abandonment, suicide; they do not even think about it; they prefer to die at home. The Lebanese who answered "yes" believe that it depends on their health; if they become dependent; not to bother the family; if they are alone. [63]

11.4.3. The need to protect the integuments

A study conducted in Benin by Mouftaou AMADOU SANNI states that the results of the 2007 CEFORP study and various other surveys show that elderly people in Benin's urban areas, particularly in the urban agglomeration of Cotonou, are subject to isolation, housing, food and nutrition problems, while they must deal with the city's complex and expensive environmental, psychosocial, economic and health problems. According to the 2007 survey, three out of ten elderly people (30.7%) live in homes that are flooded during rainy weather; 12% of those surveyed are close to the illegal dumps that pollute their environment; and, 16% of them live in rented accommodation and face rents and all forms of humiliation from the owners. [64]

11.5. Types of housing referrals expressed by seniors.

According to Bertrand Alain in his study on the accommodation of elderly people in foster homes, he shows that the decision to choose this type of accommodation and housing is motivated by loneliness and/or by the appearance of a pathology causing dependence and therefore too much care. This decision is rarely made by the elderly themselves, but by their families, who see this solution as an extension of their previous home. According to this survey, the people cared for can be divided into three relatively balanced dependency groups (autonomous: 30%, semi-dependent: 32%, dependent: 38%). Among the dependent population, it should be noted that those suffering from psychological disorders benefit from a more thorough medical follow-up and periods of hospitalization to overcome periods of crisis. In addition, foster families benefit from more psychological support. [65]

11.5.1. Social and psychological assistance for the elderly

In an article entitled "Living conditions and vulnerability of the elderly", Ether Chrystelle EYINGA DIMI says that there are charitable associations, charitable NGOs that also provide support to the elderly. They offer shelter, food, material and moral assistance and educational support to the elderly. For the moment, their number is still quite limited. Naturally, they receive room and board,

---

[63] Nicole CAMPUIS LUCCIANI et al, *Perception de la prise en charge des personnes de troisième âge de libanaises, marocaines et sénégalaises* in Vieillissement de la population dans les pays du sud, Art, université de cheikh Anta Diope, Sénégal, mars 2011

[64] Mouftaou AMADOU SANNI, *Les défis urbains de vieillissement au Benin*, in Vieillissement de la population dans les pays du sud CEFORP, May 2011.

[65] Bertrand Alain, *Hébergement des personnes âgées en famille d'accueil*, dissertation (unpublished), Institut supérieur de formation en soins infirmiers de Verdun, 1995-1998, p13.

in short a social assistance allowing them to continue to live much better than outside this framework. [66]

11.5.2. Family assistance for the elderly

Nicole CAMPUIS LUCCIANI et al in a comparative study on the perception of the care of elderly Lebanese, Moroccans and Senegalese, states that the majority of Moroccans and Senegalese want home help; especially Moroccans living in France who want home help, provided that it is free. As for the Lebanese, the majority said "no" because they felt they could still manage on their own, or with the help of their family. Some said they wanted to remain in control of their own homes; others felt handicapped if they needed outside assistance. Those who answered "yes" mentioned fatigue, the need for age, illness, but also being able to rely on someone. Note that the Lebanese living in Senegal all have a domestic help. The same reasons were given by the Senegalese and Moroccans: the younger members of the family help them; they feel autonomous; they would like help because they have no strength left but do not have the financial means to hire a professional assistant. The vast majority of the Senegalese interviewed felt that they could count on someone in case of a hard time, regardless of where they lived. The same is true for Moroccans, except when they live in France where they feel little support; 65% of them feel they can only count on themselves or rely on God. [67]

The majority of support remains family-based (first the children, then the spouse, brothers and sisters) regardless of the country. Friends and neighbors also appear, especially for Senegalese living in France and for Lebanese, as friends seem to take over from distant family. Moroccans and Senegalese living in France also mention institutional help, that of the social worker. [68]

11.5.3. Medical care

According to Ahou Clémentine TANOH in her study cited above, it shows that the elderly cared for in institutions are less and less numerous, because they are placed there in a prolonged way at an increasingly advanced age. Nearly two-thirds of those over 65 live in cities or urban communities. But in the countryside, the proportion of retired people is much higher than that of retired city dwellers. [69]

---

[66] Esther Chrystelle EYINGA DIMI, *Living conditions and vulnerability of the elderly in the South, Socio-economic situations of the elderly in Cameroon*, Art, op cit.
[67] Nicole CAMPUIS LUCCIANI et al, *perception de la prise en charge des personnes de troisième âge de libanaises, marocaines et sénégalaises*, op cit.
[68] Id.
[69] Ahou Clémentine TANOH, *Etude sur les conditions de vie des personnes âgées en côte d'Ivoire*: Regard sur la maltraitance à Adjame Village, op cit.

In Algeria, after independence, the main health programs gave priority to the fight against infant mortality and communicable diseases, then to fertility control and maternal protection. The social category represented by people over 60 years of age has always been integrated into the adult population at the family, social, economic and medical levels. Their low representation in the overall population has meant that this section of society has never benefited from a specific medico-social or health policy for old age. This has favored and forced these people to live with their families. The gerontological policy in Algeria is still in its infancy, and there is an almost total absence of measures and devices to deal with the problems related to old age and loss of autonomy. [70]

11.5.4. Economic Assistance

Ira Bruno (2006) also conducted a study on the living conditions of the elderly under the title: Living conditions of the elderly and social and family solidarity in the face of poverty in urban areas: the case of the city of Abidjan. According to him, since the beginning of the 1980s, when the socio-economic crisis directly affected the livelihoods of the population, the social category of the elderly has become increasingly vulnerable to poverty. To this end, it shows that the number of elderly people living below the poverty line, which is 183,358 CFA francs per person per year, is increasing. Also, poor households headed by the elderly have increased in less than two decades, from 11 percent of the population in 1985 to 36 percent in 2002. Unlike the elderly in Finland who benefit from social housing rehabilitated and equipped by the State, 36.99% of the elderly in Côte d'Ivoire in general and Abidjan in particular are tenants of the houses they live in and 6.69% are housed by their families. [71]

11.6. Summary of the literature review

After reading the results and the literature of different studies on the needs related to the establishment of old people's homes in different environments, it is worthwhile to summarize that these studies show that old people's homes or nursing homes have been created late in Africa and especially in developing countries while the new initiative of social protection of the elderly beats record in the European or Western countries. This is a more advanced culture and allows a longer life span for this vulnerable population. However, in spite of the difficulties that the elderly are experiencing within their families and in the homes for the elderly, the forms of abuse, the housing conditions and the housing that are harmful to health are increasingly proven in the different previous studies that we have referred to. These studies unfortunately show that few African countries have a culture of protection for the elderly. Many elderly people prefer to stay in the family and especially in the office environment as the elderly like to smoke.

---

[70] OUAHIBA Benalla et al, Old age in the South, comparative approaches, *What is the place of third age people in loss of autonomy*, Art, University of Bouira, Algeria, March 2011.

[71] Ira bruno, *Conditions de vie des personnes âgées et solidarité sociale et familiale à l'épreuve de la pauvreté en milieu urbain, (unpublished)*, Thesis, Abidjan 2007.

11.7. Research Frameworks

It is worth noting that the diagram we present below directly visualizes or shows the themes emerging from the present study (conceptual framework), the independent variables as well as the dependent variable to which we will go into more detail (operational framework).

11.7.1. Conceptual framework
Independent   variablesDependent variables

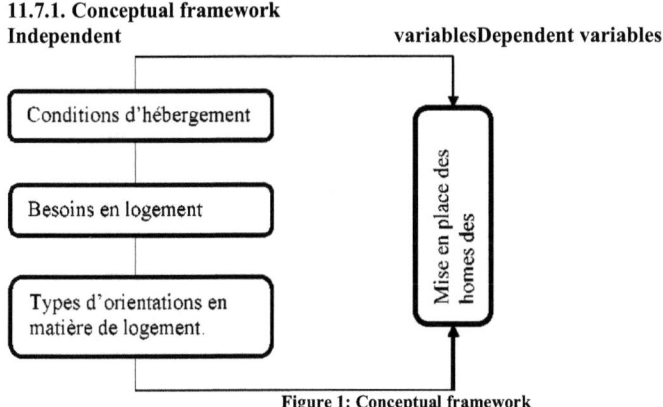

Figure 1: Conceptual framework

11.7.2. Operational framework

Independent variables   **Dependent variables**

- **Conditions d'hébergement**
  - L'insécurité alimentaire ;
  - Maltraitances psychophysiques ;
  - Déconsidération au sein de leurs familles ;
  - Faible contribution financière.

- **Besoins en logement**
  - Les locaux adaptés à leurs conditions physiques ;
  - Le souhait d'habiter le home ;
  - Besoins de protéger leurs téguments.

- **Types d'orientations en matière de logement**
  - L'Assistance sociale ;
  - Aides familiales ;
  - Accompagnement psychologique ;
  - Prise en charge médicale ;
  - Assistance économique.

Mise en place des homes des vieillards

11.7. Operational definition of variables

We define here some variables that, in the context of the present work, may be outside the usual context. The different definitions below are contextual to the present work.

❖ Independent variables

1. **Food insecurity:** By food insecurity, we mean the lack of quantity and quality of food for the health and survival of the elderly. This can be nutritional and can lead to the rapid death of the elderly.
2. **Psycho-physical abuse:** This refers to harmful acts and offensive words addressed to the elderly within or outside their families in the form of threats and which may cause stress or other psychological disorders in the elderly. These abuses can be beatings, slaps and blackmail.
3. **Disregard within the family:** Here it is a question of the place the elderly person occupies in the family and how the children and other family members behave towards the elderly person.
4. **Low financial contribution:** Being able to provide a contribution within the family for a care while taking into account its reviewed either if it is retired.
5. **Premises adapted to their physical conditions:** Often the old people are exposed to difficult practices by the premises, that is to say all the instruments and materials of the household or outside putting the old people at ease in order to survive better.
6. **Desire to live in the home:** It is the desire to leave the household or family and go to a place where the elderly can receive the social protection that medical for a long life expectancy.
7. **Needs to protect their integuments:** Some old people have the wish and desire to live in the city, in an environment where the environment allows them to protect the integuments in order to provide even more strength to meet their needs.
8. **Social assistance:** It is the whole of the goods and services granted in favor of the old people for its protection and its survival.
9. **Family assistance:** This is the set of goods and services from different families to enhance the daily life of the elderly.
10. **Psychological accompaniment:** In the conception of this study, the psychological accompaniment states all the activities that can arouse a favorable morality to the old people either to de-stress him and to forget certain harmful situations posed in his respect.
11. **Medical care:** With regard to the medical care of the elderly, all forms of medical activities (promotional, preventive and curative) carried out for the elderly.
12. **Economic assistance:** Here, it is a question of making a financial contribution, or forming IGAs for the self-care of the elderly.

❖ Dependent variable

Establishment of homes for the elderly

In the conception of this work, it is necessary to understand by homes of old people, the whole of the infrastructures or houses that can inhabit the old people for a social, psychological so much medical protection.

Chapter Three.
METHODOLOGICAL APPROACH OF THE STUDY

111.1. Introduction

This chapter presents the way we proceeded to collect data in the field, defining the type of study, the study population, the target population, the determination of the sample size, the type of sampling, the methods, techniques and tools for data collection, the recruitment, selection and training of interviewers, the pre-test, the conduct of the survey itself, the data entry, processing and analysis, ethical considerations including difficulties encountered in the field.

111.2. Type of study

The present study is of the evaluative and transversal type; it is evaluative by the fact that it allowed us to assess the needs on the establishment of old people's homes in the health zone of Goma. This study is cross-sectional because it is limited to a specific period of time, with research beginning in February 2014 and ending in July 2014. Thus, to collect data in the field, we used the quantitative approach because it allowed us to collect numerical data through a survey questionnaire of the closed type and the qualitative approach that allowed us to collect data not quantified from key informants.

111.3. Study population

For this study, the study population includes all elderly people in the Goma health zone, which is estimated to be 19586 elderly people according to the 2013 report. [72]

111.4. Target population

The target population, also known as the parent population, is made up of the elderly population, i.e., people in the 65 to 85+ age group in the Goma zone, which numbered 8061 elderly people in 2013. [73]

111.5. Sampling

In this section we will determine the sample size and the type of sampling we used to collect the data in the field. The sampling is of the probabilistic type in order to offer the chance to all the old people to be selected.

---

[72] Bureau de l'état civil, commune de Goma, census report by age group, 2013.
[73] Id.

II.4.1. Determination of the sample size

To determine the sample size we used the formula of LYNCH followed the strata sampling method because the Goma health zone consists of nine health areas. It should be noted that these nine health areas were considered as nine strata to manipulate this type of sampling. In addition, the qualitative information from the three key informants (household heads) complemented the information provided by all elderly people in the Goma health zone within their households. Thus, the lynch formula is as follows[74]

$$n = \frac{NZ^2 p(1-p)}{Nd^2 + Z^2 p(1-p)}$$

Where n= The sample size

N= Population size (Number of elderly people aged 65 to 85 and over in the Goma health zone, which is equal to 8061 elderly people in 2013) [75]

P= The prevalence or crude mortality rate among the elderly which is 11% for the year 2012-2013. [76]

$$n = \frac{8061(1,96)^2 \times 0,11(1-0,11)}{8061(0,05)^2 + (1,96)^2 \times 0,11(1-0,11)} = \frac{8061 \times 3,8416 \times 0,0979}{8061(0,0025) + 3,84 \times 0,0979}$$

$$= \frac{8061 \times 0,37609}{20,1525 + 0,37609} = \frac{3031,6827}{21,5285} = 140,82 = 141 \text{ vieillards}$$

11.4.2. Type of sampling

To carry out this research, we used stratified sampling as described in the previous paragraph. The latter, through the principle of use of this type of sampling, allowed us to survey the population on the basis of size in each health area.

---

[74] NTABE NAMAGABE Edmond, *course in action research,* (unpublished), ULPGL/GOMA ,2011-2012.
[75] Goma Health Zone Central Office, *Annual Report*, 2012, op cit.
[76] Id.

Table 3: Calculation of stratified sampling[77]

No	Health areas	Workforce old people/AS/2013	Households	Proportion	Older people to	No survey
01	CASOP	2117	302	0,11	15	57
02	MAPENDO	2521	360	0,13	18	57
03	HIMBI	1135	162	0,058	9	57
04	KATINDO	1525	218	0,08	11	57
05	HEAL AFRICA	2442	349	0,12	17	57
06	CARMEL	2257	322	0,11	16	57
07	KYESHERO	3298	471	0,17	24	57
08	CCLK	3176	454	0,16	23	57
09	BUHIMBA	1115	159	0,06	8	57
	TOTAL	19586	2797	1	141	

To calculate :

J Household= Pop/7 ;

J Proportion = Number/Total elderly

J Number of elderly to be surveyed per stratum = n (sample) x Proportion

S *Given that* N is equal to 8061, the sampling step = N (Total Pop) / n (sample).

III.5. Procedure of the investigation
111.5.1. Recruitment, selection and training of investigators

In order to collect data for this study, five headmen from the Goma health zone were recruited as interviewers, as they had a better understanding of the purpose of the training they had undergone and had a good understanding of the geographical area of the Goma health zone. These interviewers were recruited, selected and trained for one day on the basis of these criteria. The training was based on the objectives of this study, the techniques for filling out the survey questionnaire, including respect for ethical considerations to be observed in the field during the actual collection of data related to this study, before deployment in the field.

111.5.2. Pre-test

The pre-test was carried out in the KARISIMBI health zone because the latter may or may not be spared from the situation of the elderly. Keep in mind that this pre-test was carried out to avoid bias in the research, i.e. on 10 elderly people in the KARISIMBI health zone, whose results allowed us to correct any errors that were made during the development of the survey questionnaire.

---

[77] NTABE NAMEGABE Edmond, cours de recherche action, (unpublished), ULPGL/GOMA, op cit.

III.5.3. Conduct of the investigation itself

The survey was conducted in the nine health areas of the health zone by five heads of avenues from the Goma health zone. The latter were divided into two chiefs per health area. It should be noted that before beginning data collection, each interviewer was provided with survey questionnaires, which allowed them to collect data in the field. The survey was conducted within a three-day period because it was sanctioned by reaching the sample size. The snowballing technique allowed the interviewers to find the elderly in their respective households. However, in order to access the qualitative data related to this study, we contacted the three people in charge of the different households in the health zone, including one from the Kyeshero neighborhood and two others from the Volcanoes neighborhood, because these two neighborhoods contain a higher number of elderly people than the others.

III.5. 4. Data entry, processing and analysis

After the quantitative data were collected, they were processed using the SPSS (Statistical package for social science) software; the data entry was done in Microsoft Word. It should be noted that the results (numerical data) are presented in the form of tables of numbers and percentages, while the qualitative data are processed manually and presented in the form of boxes.

III.5.5. Inclusion and exclusion criteria

Being part of the survey was no accident. We were guided by the following criteria:
- To be a senior citizen from and living in the health zone of Goma;
- Be a person in the age range of 65 to 85 and over;
- Only people in the health zone under consideration were included in the survey,
- Have lived in this health zone for more than 5 years to be likely to provide quality and truthful information.
- However, all other persons not in the health zone or health area and not having a considerable duration in the setting were excluded from this survey.

III.6. Evaluation criteria
01. Criteria for assessing the needs related to the housing conditions of third age people.

Criterion 1: Reported that the housing conditions in their households are good;

Criterion 2: Reported poor housing conditions in their households;

Third criterion: Specify cassava or maize foufou as the usual food to be taken in their household;

Fourth criterion: Specify beans, fish and vegetables as the usual foods to take in their households;

Fifth criterion: Specify that they eat once or twice a day in their households;

Sixth criterion: Claimed to have experienced physical abuse in their families; **Seventh criterion:** Denied having ever experienced physical abuse in their families; **Eighth criterion:** Specified slapping or hitting as physical abuse in their families;

Ninth criterion: Specify deliberate harassment and injury as physical abuse already experienced

within the family;
Tenth criterion: have admitted to ever having experienced psychological abuse within their families;
Criterion 11: Denied ever experiencing emotional abuse in their families;
Criterion 12: Stated that they are consulted when decisions are made within their families;
Thirteenth criterion: Deny that they are consulted when decisions are made within their families;
Fourteenth criterion: Specify that they are not considered in the decision making in their respective families because of the advanced age;
Instructions or Prerequisites:

- *S* Responded favorably to the criteria 1st, 4th, 7th, 11th and 12th: ***Good accommodation conditions.***
- S Answered favorably to criteria 2nd, 3rd, 5th, 6th, 8th, 9th, 10th, 13th and 14th: ***Poor housing conditions.***

02. Criteria for assessing the needs related to the housing conditions of the elderly First criterion: Specify the durable material as the type of housing they live in; **Second criterion:** Specify the plank house as the type of housing they live in; **Third criterion:** Affirm that the house they live in allows them to make all physical movements;
Fourth criterion: Deny that the house they live in allows them to make any physical movement;
Fifth criterion: Claim that the house they live in is served by water and electricity; **Sixth criterion:** Deny that the house they live in is served by water and electricity; **Seventh criterion:** Specify the single pit latrine as the type of latrine used;
Eighth criterion: Specify septic tank latrine as the type of latrine used **Ninth criterion:** Specify that the latrine used is maintained once or twice a week. **Tenth criterion:** Confessed to having heard of an old people's home;
Criterion 11: Denied ever having heard of old people's homes
Twelfth criterion: Have stated that they wish to live in a retirement home for the rest of their lives;
Thirteenth criterion: Deny that they want to live in a retirement home for the rest of their lives;
Instructions or Prerequisites:

- *S* Answered favorably to the criteria 1st, 3rd, 5th, 9th, 10th, i and 12th: ***Good housing conditions.***
- S Responded favorably to the 2nd, 4th, 6th, 7th, 8th, and 13th criteria: ***Poor housing conditions.***

03. Evaluation criteria related to the types of referrals expressed by the elderly
Criterion 1: Claim to have ever received social assistance from outside the family; **Criterion 2:** Deny having ever received social assistance from outside the family; **Criterion 3:** Wish to receive assistance from within the family;

Fourth criterion: Do not want help from family;

Fifth criterion: Claim to have ever suffered from an illness;

Sixth criterion: Deny ever having had an illness;

Seventh criterion: Specify self-medication or use of traditional medicinal plants as types of care received during illness

Criterion Eight: Desire special medical assistance in case of illness;

Ninth criterion: Do not want medical assistance in case of illness;
Tenth criterion: Have a desire to receive economic assistance to support themselves;

Criterion 11: Do not have a desire to receive economic assistance to support themselves;

Instructions or Prerequisites:

S Responded favorably to criteria 1st, 3rd, 5th, 8th, and 10th: *Good types of orientations.*

S Responded favorably to criteria 2nd, 4th, 6th, 7th, 9th and 11th: *Wrong types of referrals.*

111.7. Data collection methods, techniques and tools

To collect the data, we used various methods, including the quantitative method, which allowed us to collect numerical data. This method was combined with the structured interview technique in the form of questioning, and a semi-closed survey questionnaire to facilitate the collection of numerical data from 141 elderly people in the Goma health zone.

In addition, the qualitative method was used to collect the views of our key informants on the needs for the establishment of the old people's homes in the Goma health zone. These were collected using an unstructured interview technique with the help of a supporting interview guide to facilitate the collection of qualitative information from three household leaders in the Goma health zone.

111.8. Ethical considerations

In order to promote research ethics, we explained to the respondents the objectives of this study. Participation in this study was neither compulsory nor imposing, but it was based on the good faith of the respondents and especially on their free or voluntary consent. We also guaranteed the confidentiality of the information received by the respondents through anonymity or the use of codes on the survey questionnaire.

111.9. Remedies

Within the framework of a vision to reach the objectives in this study, at the end of this one, recommendations were addressed to the targets, this in order to be able to concretize the real needs expressed by the target for the establishment of the old people's homes.

111.10. Dissemination of results

This study needs to be made available for dissemination so that the results reach those who really need them. This is primarily the central office of the
Goma health zone, who respectively stated that they needed data on third age people.

Nevertheless, this study must be made accessible to all the other ambitious researchers who have the desire to get to know the reality of the care of third age people from the results of this work.

111.11.   Difficulties encountered :

A scientific work never lacks difficulties. After the survey itself and during the data processing, we came up against certain constraints or difficulties that did not allow us to move forward. This is why the major difficulty we experienced was the loss of nine protocols after the survey, which forced us to return to the field. In addition, the fatigue of some elderly people to answer the questions during the questioning stage.

Chapter Four.
PRESENTATION AND INTERPRETATION OF RESULTS
IV.0. Introduction

In this chapter, after data analysis, we present the results in accordance with our initial objectives. Thus, we describe the results concerning the characteristics of the respondents, the housing conditions of the elderly, the housing needs experienced by the elderly and the types of housing referrals expressed by the elderly. **IV.1 Characteristics of respondents**

Q01. Age du répondant

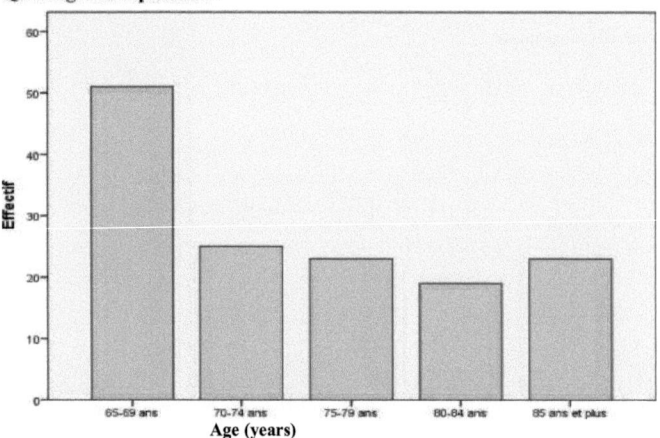

Figure 1: Distribution of respondents by age

The results presented in this bar graph show that among the 141 old people to be surveyed, 51 respondents or 36.2% were in the 65-69 age group, while those aged 70-74 constitute 25 respondents or 17.7%, but also 23 respondents or 16.3% are in the 75-79 age group. At the same time, 23 and 19 (16.3% and 13.5%) are aged 84 and over and 80-84 respectively. This shows that the older old people surveyed are less numerous than those who are still close to adulthood. This explains why the older they get, the fewer they are in the Goma health zone.

Q02. Gender of respondent

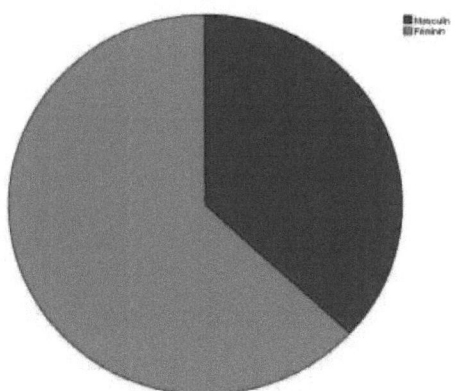

Figure 2: Distribution of respondents by gender

The results presented in this sector graph show that old women are represented by the color green and occupy a higher proportion than men in the sample with 89 respondents, i.e. 63.1% more than men who are represented by the color blue with 52 respondents, i.e. 36.9%. **Q03. What is your level of education?**

Table 4: Distribution of respondents by level of education

Level of study	Workforce	%
Primary completed	19	13.5
Primary not completed	26	18.4
Secondary completed	24	17
Secondary not completed	21	14.9
University completed	3	2.1
University not completed	4	2.8
No level of education	44	31.2
Total	**141**	**100**

The results that fill this table show that out of a sample of 141 respondents, a proportion of 31.2% have no level of education, 18.4% of respondents have not completed primary education, 17% of respondents have completed secondary education against 14.9% of respondents who have not completed secondary education, 13.5% have attended elementary school up to the 6th grade and have obtained the certificate of completion of primary education, but also a minority, 2.8% have not completed higher education against another minority, 2.1% who have completed university.

A minority of 2.8% did not complete higher education and another minority of 2.1% completed university. This shows that the elderly in the Goma Health Zone have a low intellectual level.

Q04. What is your religious affiliation?

Table 5: Distribution of respondents by religious denomination.

Religious denomination	Staffing	%
Catholic	60	42.6
Protestant	56	39.7
Muslim	7	5
Jehova's Witness	2	1.4
Revival Church	5	3.5
Adventist	2	1.4
Neo Apostolic	9	6.4
Total	**141**	**100**

The observation of this table allows us to see that almost half, or 42.6% of the elderly are Catholics, 39.7% are Protestants, followed by a minority, or 6.4%, who are of the New Apostolic faith and 5% are Muslims. But also, 3.5% of the elderly attend revivalist churches. Finally, Jehova's Witnesses and Adventists represent the same proportion of 1.4%.

Q05. What is your marital status?

Table 6: Distribution of respondents by marital status.

Marital status	Staffing	%
Single	2	1.4
Married	58	41.1
Widow(er)	71	50.4
Divorced	9	6.4
United in fact	1	0.7
Total	**141**	**100**

It appears from this table that half of the respondents, i.e. 50.4%, are widows, almost half, i.e. 41.1%, are married and 6.4% are divorced. Finally, single elderly people and de facto unions represent a very small proportion, respectively 1.4% and 0.7% of the sample.

IV.2 Accommodation conditions for the elderly

Q06. How are the living arrangements in your household?

Table 7: Appreciation of housing conditions in households.

Appreciations	Workforce	%
Very good	5	3.5
Good	81	57.5
Fairly good	37	26.3
Bad	13	9.2
Very bad	3	2.1
Poor	2	1.4
Total	**141**	**100**

As one would expect, table 07 indicates that more than half, or 57.5% of the subjects, live in good housing conditions, 26.3% say that the conditions are fairly good, while a minority, 9.2%, say that they have poor conditions. Similarly, those who live in very good conditions represent 3.5%. A very low proportion of 2.1% and 1.4% of respondents say that they live in very bad and poor housing conditions.

Q07. What food do you usually eat?

Table 8: Distribution of respondents by usual food types

Types of food	Workforce	%
Foufou of manioc or corn	53	37.6
Beans and Rice	22	15.6
Fish	19	13.5
Vegetables and fruits	34	24.1
Everything I find I take	11	7.8
Meat	2	1.4
Total	**141**	**100**

The table shows that only 37.6% of respondents eat cassava or corn, 24.1% eat vegetables and fruit, and those who are used to eating beans and rice represent 15.6%, compared to 13.5% who eat fish. Similarly, a minority, 7.8%, eat whatever they can find, and 1.4% are used to eating meat. This leads us to say that the elderly in the Goma Health Zone are more accustomed to taking protective foods.

Q08. How often do you eat per day?

Table 9: Number of times per day to take the meal

Number of times	Workforce	%
Once a day	18	12.8
Twice a day	66	46.8
Three times a day	36	25.5
More than three times/day	20	14.2
Depending on availability	1	0.7
Total	**141**	**100**

In the light of this table, it appears from these results that almost half, i.e. 46.8%, take the meal twice a day, followed by 25.5% who do so three times a day. Those who eat more than three times a day represent a proportion of 14.2% compared to those who eat once a day who occupy a proportion of 12.8% and finally an old man or 0.7% who said that he eats according to the availability of food.

Q09. Have you ever been physically abused in your family or elsewhere?

Table 10: Physical abuse suffered by the elderly within the family or elsewhere

Answer	Workforce	%
Yes	56	39.7
No	85	60.3
Total	**141**	**100**

The results of this table show that 85 respondents (60.3%) denied that they had ever been physically abused in their families or elsewhere, compared to 56 respondents (39.7%) who said they had been physically abused.

Q10. If yes, which one?

Table 11: Types of physical abuse experienced by the watchers within their families or elsewhere.

Type of physical abuse	Workforce	%
Slap or blow	13	23.2
Harassment	18	32.1
Untreated or poorly treated pressure sores	14	25
Brutality	7	12.5
Deliberate injury	4	7.1
Total	**56**	**100**

The observation of this table lets us see that out of the number of respondents who affirmed to have already undergone physical abuse, 32.1% talk about having already undergone harassment, 23.2% of the respondents specify the slap or blow put on them within the family or elsewhere, 25% talk about the persistence of untreated or poorly treated bedsores, 12.5% talk about brutality and 7.1% have already undergone deliberate injuries.

Q11. Have you ever experienced emotional abuse in your family or elsewhere?

Table 12: Psychological abuse suffered by the elderly within the family or elsewhere

Answer	Workforce	%
Yes	89	63.1
No	52	36.9
Total	**141**	**100**

The results of this table show that 89 respondents, or more than half (63.1%), said that they had already been psychologically abused within their respective families or elsewhere, compared to 52 respondents (36.9%) who denied having ever been psychologically abused.

Q12. if yes, which one?

Table 13: Types of psychological abuse suffered by the watchers within their families or elsewhere.

Psychological abuse	Workforce	%
Insult	25	28.1
Shocking words	28	31.5
Humiliation	19	21.3
I am stressed	17	19.1
Total	**89**	**100**

The elements of this table let us see that among the respondents who affirmed to have undergone a psychological mistreatment towards them, 31,5% speak about having already received shocking words addressed to them, 28,1% of the respondents speak about insults made towards them within the family or elsewhere, 21,3% evoke humiliation, 19,1% say that they are stressed at any moment.

Q13. When making decisions within the family, are you consulted?

Tableau 14: consultation of the elderly in family decision making.

Answer	Workforce	%
Yes	102	72.3
No	39	27.7
Total	**141**	**100**

In view of this table, it is important to note that the majority of respondents (72.3%) claim to have been consulted in the decision-making process within their respective host families, while 27.7% deny or say the opposite.

Q14. If yes, are your views taken into account?

Tableau 15: Level of consideration of point of view when making decisions in the family.

Consideration	Workforce	%
Not quite	13	12.7
Sometimes	44	43.2
Partially	20	19.6
Totally	25	24.5
Total	**102**	**100**

In light of this table, we note that among the respondents who said they are consulted before the decision is made in their respective families, nearly half, i.e. 43.2%, say they are consulted some of the time, 24.5% are consulted totally, those who are partially consulted occupy 19.6% against 12.7% who say they are consulted but not completely.

Q15. If not, why not?

Table 16: Reasons for not taking into account the family's point of view when making decisions

Reasons	Workforce	%
I am not considered to be at fault for advanced	4	10.3
I am neglected	22	56.4
I am considered a child	12	30.8
I don't stay next to my family anymore	1	2.6
Total	39	100

Among the respondents who denied being consulted by their families when making decisions, more than half (56.4%) gave a reason of being neglected by the family, 30.8% said that they were considered a child in the family. Likewise, 10.3% said that they were not considered because of their advanced age and 2.6% gave the reason that they did not stay with the family.

Q16. What is your occupation?

Table 17: Distribution of respondents by type of occupation

Types of occupations	Staffing	%.
Trader	20	14.2
State employee	14	9.9
Cultivator	10	7.1
Retired	29	20.6
Unemployed or unemployed	56	39.7
Trade	12	8.5
Total	141	100

With regard to the results of this table, we note that most of the respondents, i.e. 39.7%, are unemployed, 20.6% are retired, 14.2% are traders and 9.9% are government employees. However, 8.5% of the respondents practice trades within their households and 7.1% practice agriculture, so they are farmers.

Q17. How much can you estimate your contribution to your household's monthly income?

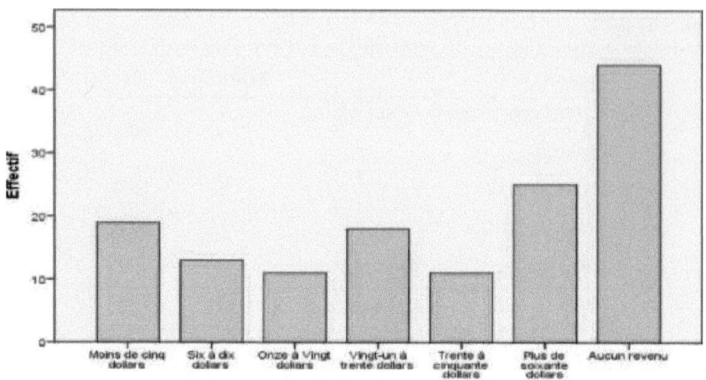

Figure 3: Distribution of the elderly by estimated monthly income

In view of this bar graph, it is worth noting that out of the total number of respondents, 44 respondents (31.2%) contribute nothing throughout the month within their families, followed by 25 respondents (17.7%) who contribute more than $60 per month, 19 respondents (13.5%) who contribute less than $5 per month. But also, 18 respondents or 12.8% contribute in the range of 20 to 30$ per month within their respective families, 13 respondents or 9.2% contribute 6 to 10$ per month. However, those who contribute between $11 to $20 and $30 to $50 represent 11 respondents or 7.8%, so they are on the same level.

Table 18: Scorecard on the evaluation of housing conditions for the elderly in the Goma health zone.

Criteria	Workforce	%
Responded favorably to the 1st, 4th, 7th, 11th and 12th criteria: *Good conditions accommodation.*	88	62,4
Responded favorably to the criteria 2nd, 3rd, 5th, 6th, 8th *Poor conditions accommodation*	53	37,6
Total	**141**	**100**

The results of this table show that out of **141** elderly people in the Goma health zone, **88** respondents **(62.4%)** responded positively to the criteria of good housing conditions, while **53** respondents **(37.6%)** indicated that housing conditions were poor. Based on the above scores, we can conclude that the housing conditions for the elderly in the Goma Health Zone are *good*.

Box 1: Interview with a head of a household with an elderly person in KYESHERO, Les Volcans and HIMBI.

When asked about the conditions in which the elderly are housed, the people in charge of the households answered that the conditions in which the elderly are housed are good; they live in frank collaboration with them, they share all together despite the little means they have, they like living with these elderly and also they owe them respect.

When they are in conditions of illness, disability and partial or total dependence, there is a specific person who takes care of them by offering accompaniment in all services/needs (bathing, eating, relief,...)

IV.3. Housing needs experienced by the elderly

Q18. What type of housing do you live in?

Table 19: Type of housing used by the elderly

Types of housing	Workforce	%
Durable material	58	41.1
Plank house	77	54.6
Tarpaulin house	4	2.8
Straw house	2	1.4
Total	141	100

In view of this table, the results show that out of a total of 141 respondents, more than half, or 58%, live in a house made of sustainable materials, followed by those who live in plank houses, or 54.6%, against a minority, or 2.8%, and 1.4% who live in houses made of tarpaulin and straw.

Q19. Does the house you live in allow for all physical movement?

Table 20: Exercise of the physical movements and the type of housing accommodated by the old

Answer	Workforce	%
Yes	76	53.9
No	65	46.1
Total	141	100

From this table, it emerges that more than half, 53.9% of the respondents, say that the house they live in allows them to exercise all the physical movement against 46.1% who say the opposite.

Q20. If not, how?

Table 21: Reasons for not exercising physical movement in the homes where the elderly live

Reasons	Workforce	%
No armchairs or adequate chairs	43	66.1
The stairs are very long	2	3.1
Humidity (cold)	11	16.9
No light	5	7.7
No space (smallness of the house)	4	6.2
Total	65	100

Among the respondents who denied that the house does not allow them to exercise all the physical movements, more than half of them, 66.1%, said that their houses do not have adequate chairs and armchairs, 16.9% said that the house is damp (cold), 7.7% said that it is because there is no light in the house (electricity), while 6.2% said that the house is too small and finally, 3.1% said that the stairs in the house are very long.

Q21. Is your home served by water and electricity?

Table 22: Availability of water and electricity in the house where the elderly live.

Response	Staff	%.
"OUï	90	638
No	5136	.2
Total	141	100

With regard to this table, more than half, 63.8%, affirm that their dwellings are served with drinking water and electricity, while 36.2% prove the opposite.

Q22. If yes, how often?

Table 23: Frequency of drinking water and electricity in the homes of the elderly.

Frequency	Workforce	%
Regularly	26	28.9
Irregularly	64	71.1
Total	90	100

Looking at the results of the table above, we can see that among those who affirmed that their dwellings have water and electricity, the majority of the respondents, 71.1%, say that water and electricity arrive in an irregular way, while 28.9% say that this service is regulated in their dwellings.

Q23. What type of latrine do you use?

Table 24: Types of latrines used by the elderly in their homes.

Types of latrines	Workforce	%
Single pit latrine	61	43.3
Septic tank latrine	47	33.3
Latrine with tank	22	15.6
Open-air latrine	11	7.8
Total	141	100.0

The results of this table reveal that 43.3% use a simple pit latrine or a borehole latrine in their households, 33.3% use a pit latrine, 15.6% use a pit latrine and 7.8% use an open pit latrine only.

Q24. How often is your latrine maintained?
Table 25: Frequency of latrine maintenance per week.

Frequency	Workforce	%
One time/s	34	24.1
Twice/s	29	20.6
Three times/s	14	9.9
Four times/s	18	12.8
More than five times/s	38	27
No time	7	5
I do not know	1	0.7
Total	141	100

The table shows that 27% of the respondents maintain their latrines more than five times a week, 24.1% only once a week, 20.6% twice a week, 12.8% four times a week, 9.9% three times a week, and 5% and 0.7% do not even do it and say they do not know.

Q25. Have you ever heard of an old people's home?
Table 26: Knowledge about the home for the elderly.

Answer	Workforce	%
Yes	41	29.1
No	100	70.9
Total	141	100

The table shows that the majority of respondents (70.9%) had heard of an old people's home, compared to 29.1% of respondents who said they had never heard of an old people's home.

Q26. Would you like to live in a nursing home for the rest of your life?
Table 27: Desire to live in a retirement home for the rest of one's life

Answer	Workforce	%
Yes	81	57.4
No	60	42.6
Total	141	100

Of the respondents, more than half (57.4%) say they want to live in the home, while 42.6% do not want to for the rest of their lives.

Q27. If yes, why

Table 28: Reasons for wanting to live in the home

Reasons	Workforce	%
I will be able to rest there	28	34.6
I will feel safer there	10	12.3
I will be well cared for there	3	3.7
My family will be relieved	13	16.1
I will meet people of my age there	27	33.3
Total	**81**	**100**

From this table, we can see that among the respondents who said that they would like to live in the home, most of them (34.6%) said that the old people's home would be a place of rest for them, 33.3% said that they would be with people of their own age, 16.1% said that it would be a relief for their family, but also 12.3% said that they would feel safer there and 3.7% said that they would be well looked after.

Q28. If not, why not?

Table 29: Reasons for not wanting to live in the home.

Reasons for not wishing	Workforce	%
I rely heavily on my children	32	53.3
It will be an abandonment	4	6.7
It's not a place of fulfillment	5	8.3
This is not our culture	19	31.7
Total	**60**	**100**

The observation of the results of this table informs us that among the respondents who do not wish to live in the home, more than half of them, 53.3%, give a reason to say that they have a lot on their children, 31.7% of them say that it is not of their culture, while 8.3% allude to a place of blooming which is not it and finally, 6.7% consider it as an abandonment of the family.

Q29. Under what conditions do you wish to live in the rest of your life?

Table 30: Desired conditions for the rest of life

Desired conditions	Workforce	%
Away from the noise	86	61
In dwellings not flooded during rainy weather	14	9.9
Housing away from polluting dumping grounds the environment	5	5.7
House without excessive cold	24	17.1
Where there is security and peace	9	6.4
Total	141	100

In view of this table, it is important to show that more than half of the respondents, 61%, say that they wish to live in conditions far from noise for the rest of their lives, 17.1% wish to live in houses without excessive cold, 9.9% want houses that are not flooded in times of rain, while 6.4% wish to live in a place where they will have more security and peace, and finally 5.7% speak of housing far from illegal dumps that pollute the environment.

Table 31: Scorecard on the evaluation of housing conditions for the elderly in the Goma Health Zone.

Criteria	Workforce	%
Answered favorably to the criteria 1st, 3rd, 5th, 9th, 10th, 11th and 12th: *Good housing conditions.*	76	54
Answered favorably to criteria 2nd, 4th, 6th, 7th, 8th and 13th: *Poor housing conditions.*	65	46
Total	141	100

The results of this table show that out of **141** elderly people in the Goma health zone, **76** respondents (**54%**) answered positively to the criteria of good housing conditions, while **65** respondents (**46%**) indicated that housing conditions were poor. Based on the above scores, we can conclude that the housing conditions of the elderly in the Goma Health Zone are *quite good.*

Box 2: Interview with a household manager with an elderly person in KYESHERO, Les Volcans and HIMBI.

When asked about the **housing needs of the elderly,** the heads of households told us that they like a well-cared for, well-ventilated, well-lit home. Some express the need to live in a house made of durable materials, well equipped and furnished, others like to live in a house made of planks because, according to them, in case of earthquake, it will be better protected.

Second, the elderly express a need to return to an environment where they will be autonomous in terms of daily control because they are under the command of the head of the household, from which they cannot act without the approval of the owner of the house who is also the head of the household.

IV.4. Types of housing orientations expressed by the elderly

Q30. Have you ever been a recipient of external social assistance

Table 32: Recipients of external social assistance.

Answer	Workforce	%
Yes	65	46.1
No	76	53.9
Total	**141**	**100**

It appears from this table that more than half, 53.9%, have already benefited from external social assistance, compared to 46.1% who have never benefited from it.

Q31. If yes, what is the source?

Table 33: Place of origin of the social assistance received.

Place of origin	Workforce	%
NGO	19	29.2
The State	7	10.8
Church	24	36.9
At my previous place of work	10	15.4
Family members	5	7.7
Total	**65**	**100**

The table above shows that among those who said they had already received social assistance, most of the respondents (36.9%) said they had received it from a church, 29.2% from an NGO, 15.5% from their previous place of work, while 10.8% had received it from the state and 7.7% from family members.

Q32. If yes, what is it about?

Table 34: Content of social assistance received.

Content	Workforce	%
Social framework	36	55.4
Practical advice	7	10.8
Counselling session	1	1.5
Cabin construction	8	12.3
Premium	3	4.6
Food	10	15.4
Total	**65**	**100**

The results of the above table show that among those who said they had ever received social assistance, more than half or 55.4% said it was social guidance, 15.4% said it was food, 12.3% had been given a hut, while 10.8% had been given practical advice while 4.6% had received bonuses from their previous workplaces and 1.5% spoke of counseling sessions.

Q33. If not, would you still like to have some?

Table 35: Desire for assistance.

Answer	Staff	%
Yes	68	89.5
No	8	10.5
Total	**76**	**100**

It is worth noting that among the respondents who have never received social assistance, a large majority (89.5%) would like to receive it anyway, even though they have not had the chance to do so, compared to 10.5% who would not.

Q34. Would you like help from your family?

Table 36: Desire for a caregiver.

Response	Staff	%.
Yes	133	94.3
No	8	5.7
Total	**141**	**100**

In the light of this table, let us note that a large proportion (94.3%) of the respondents wish to have help from their respective families against a minority (5.7%) who do not.

Q35. If yes, how

Table 37: What we want to come out of the family.

Wish	Workforce	%
I would like my family to visit me regularly	67	50.8
By meeting my basic needs	65	49.2
Total	132	100

In view of this table, it is good to prove that among those who said they wanted family assistance, half of them, i.e. 50.8%, wanted regular visits from their families, while 49.2% wanted a response to their basic needs.

Q36. If not, why not?

Table 38: Reasons for not wanting family assistance

Staff Reasons %.		
I am self-sufficient	1	11.1
I tend to the end of my life	2	22.2
I don't want to hurt my family	6	66.7
Total	9	100

In view of this table, it is worth noting that among those who deny having the desire for family assistance, more than half, 66.7%, say that they do not want to cause their families to suffer, while 22.2% say that they tend towards the end of their lives while 11.1% say that they are self-sufficient.

Q37. Have you ever suffered from an illness?

Table 39: Suffering or not from a disease

Answer	Workforce	%
Yes	137	97.2
No	4	2.8
Total	141	100

In view of this, we note that a large majority (97.2%) have already suffered from an illness in their daily lives, while a minority (2.3%) say they have never suffered from an illness.

Q38. If yes, how were you cared for?

Table 40: Place of recourse during illness.

Court	Workforce	%
Self-medication/use of medicinal plants traditional	52	38
I went to the hospital	82	59.8
Prayer only	3	2.2
Total	**137**	**100**

The results of this table show that among those who said they had already suffered from an illness, more than half, i.e. 59.8%, resorted to hospital treatment, 38% resorted to self-medication and the use of medical herbs, while 2.2% relied only on prayer.

Q39. Would you like special medical assistance in case of illness?

Table 41: Desire for medical assistance.

Answer	Workforce	%
Yes	132	93.6
No	9	6.4
Total	**141**	**100**

Of the total sample size of 141, a large majority (93.6%) of respondents wanted specialized medical assistance in case of illness, while a minority (6.4%) did not.

Q40. Do you have a desire to receive economic assistance to support yourself?

Table 42: Expressed need for economic assistance

Answer	Workforce	%
Yes	130	92.2
No	11	7.8
Total	**141**	**100**

The table shows that a large majority (92.2%) would like to receive economic assistance to meet their needs, while a minority (7.8%) would not.

Q41. If yes, what type?

Table 43: Type of economic assistance expressed

Type of assistance	Workforce	%
In kind	23	17.7
In cash	67	51.5
By AGR	40	30.8
Total	**130**	**100**

Among the respondents who expressed the desire to receive economic assistance to meet their needs, 67 respondents (51.5%) expressed the desire to receive this assistance in cash, then 40 respondents (30.8%) wanted this assistance through the opening of an income-generating activity and finally, 23 respondents (17.7%) wanted to receive economic assistance in kind.

Table 44: Score table on the evaluation of referral types expressed by elderly people in the Goma health zone.

Criteria	Staff	%
Responded favorably to criteria 1st, 3rd, 5th, 8th and 10th: *Good types of orientations.*	103	73
Responded favorably to 2nd, 4th, 6th, 7th, 9th and 11th criteria: *Bad types orientations.*	**38**	27
Total	**141**	**100**

The results from this table show that out of **141** elderly people in the Goma health zone, **103** respondents **(73%)** answered favorably to the criteria of good orientation types, while 38 respondents **(27%)** revealed the opposite. Based on the above scores, we can conclude that the types of referrals among the elderly in the Goma Health Zone are ***good and they want to stay in the home for the rest of their lives.***

**Box 3: Interview with a head of a household with an elderly person in
KYESHERO, Les Volcans and HIMBI**

To the question of what **types of orientations** are **expressed by the elderly,** the heads of households answered that they want to live in the city where they will no longer work in the fields, i.e., they want a rest. They want to live in a group to exchange ideas and comment on their past, present and even their future life. But they still rely on the present.

The most ardent wish that animates them is to live in rest without getting tired.

Chapter Five.
DISCUSSION OF THE RESULTS

V.0. Introduction

In this chapter, we will discuss the results of the present study in comparison with previous studies and theories regarding the hypotheses put forward in view of the objective of this work, which is to assess the needs for the establishment of old people's homes experienced by the elderly in the health zone of Goma.

Indeed, the discussion of the results focuses on the following points:

> Respondent Characteristics;
> Accommodation conditions for 3rd age people;
> Housing Needs Experienced by Seniors;
> Types of housing orientations expressed by seniors.

V.1 Characteristics of respondents

The sample consisted of 141 elderly people, i.e., 100%, of whom 51 respondents, i.e., 36.2%, were in the 65-69 age group, while those in the 70-74 age group constituted 25 respondents, i.e., 17.7%, and 23 respondents, i.e., 16.3%, were in the 75-79 age group. At the same time, 23 and 19 (16.3% and 13.5%) are aged 84 and over and 80-84 respectively. This shows that the older old people surveyed are less numerous than those who are still close to adulthood. This explains why the older they get, the fewer they are in the Goma health zone. The results of this study show that women outnumber men in the sample, with 89 respondents (63.1%), compared to men, who had 52 respondents (36.9%).

The results of this study show that out of a sample of 141 respondents, 31.2% have no level of education, 18.4% of respondents have not completed primary school, 17% of respondents have completed secondary school compared to 14,9% of the respondents have not completed secondary school, 13.5% have completed elementary school up to the 6th grade and have obtained the primary school leaving certificate, and a minority, 2.8%, have not completed higher education, while another minority, 2.1%, have completed university. This shows that the elderly in the Goma Health Zone have a low intellectual level.

The results of this same study show that almost half, or 42.6% of the elderly are Catholics, 39.7% are Protestants, followed by a minority, or 6.4%, who are of the New Apostolic faith and 5% are Muslims. But also, 3.5% of the elderly attend revivalist churches. Finally, Jehova's Witnesses and Adventists represent the same proportion, i.e. 1.4%. It appears from this study that half of the respondents, i.e. 50.4%, are widows, almost half, i.e. 41.1%, are married and 6.4% are divorced. Finally, single elderly people and de facto unions represent a very small proportion, respectively 1.4% and 0.7% of the sample.

V.2 Accommodation conditions for the elderly

In observing the hypothesis that food insecurity, psycho-physical maltreatment, low esteem within their families, and low financial contribution would be the housing conditions of the elderly in the health zone of Goma, the results of this study show that more than half, or 57.5% of the subjects live in good housing conditions, 26.3% say that the conditions are fairly good, while a minority say that the conditions are bad. Similarly, those who live in very good conditions represent 3.5%. A very low proportion of 2.1% and 1.4% of the respondents say that they live in very bad and poor accommodation conditions.

In the same study, speaking of the type of food, it was found that only 37.6% of respondents eat cassava or corn, 24.1% eat vegetables and fruit, and those who are used to eating beans and rice represent 15.6% against 13.5% who eat fish. Similarly, a minority, 7.8%, eat whatever they can find, and 1.4% are used to eating meat. This leads us to say that the elderly in the Goma Health Zone are more accustomed to taking protective foods. From these results, we can see that almost half (46.8%) eat twice a day followed by 25.5% who eat three times a day. Those who eat more than three times a day represent a proportion of 14.2% compared to those who eat once a day who occupy a proportion of 12.8% and finally an old man or 0.7% who said that he eats according to the availability of food.

These results differ from those obtained by Ahou Clémentine TANOH in her study on the living conditions of the elderly in Côte d'Ivoire who testify that the social elders of Adjamé-village, according to their culture, eat essentially attiéké (Agbodjama) made with cassava, but also foutou or foufou (cocotcha) of yam or plantain. These dishes are accompanied by "clear" sauce, "seed" sauce or "N'tro" sauce with "good" fish specific to the lagoons such as broché, machoiron, captain,
They are fished directly in the lagoon. However, with the current pollution of the lagoon, fishing is no longer practiced by the villagers. [78]

Partially we can conclude by saying that the choice of food to be consumed regularly by the old people depends on the culture of the environment in which he lives, the availability of food and the income of the family that supports him.

Concerning the types of abuse suffered by the elderly within their families or elsewhere, the results of this study show that 85 respondents (60.3%) deny that they have ever been physically abused within their respective families or elsewhere, compared to 56 respondents (39.7%) who claim to have already suffered this act of physical abuse. Of the respondents who said they had already suffered physical abuse, 32.1% said they had already been harassed, 23.2% of the respondents said they had been slapped or hit within the family or elsewhere, 25% said they had suffered from untreated or poorly treated bedsores, 12.5% said they had been beaten and 7.1% had already suffered deliberate injury. In the same study, 89 respondents (63.1%) stated that they had already been psychologically abused by their families or elsewhere, compared to 52 respondents (36.9%) who denied having ever been psychologically abused. Among the respondents who said they had been psychologically abused, 31.5% said they had been insulted, 28.1% said they had been insulted within the family or elsewhere and/or in institutions, 21.3% said they had been humiliated, and 19.1% said they were under constant stress.

Our results are similar to those obtained by Robert Hugonot and Françoise Busby quoted by Ahou Clémentine TANOH who state that the elderly are mistreated both in the family and in institutions. In both cases, several categories of abuse are noted. The most frequent forms of abuse are financial and psychological (27% each). In the financial area, it is not only the withholding of pensions, thefts, swindles, anticipated inheritance, robbery of money, movable and immovable goods, but also living off the grandparents. Physical abuse (15% of the reported cases) includes beatings, slaps, and untreated or badly treated bedsores. Less known than the previous ones, but very numerous (15%) are the neglects of daily life assistance, voluntary or not: getting up, going to bed, washing, eating, walking. To these must be added murder, deliberate assault and battery, rape, tying to a bed or chair, inadequate feeding, etc. Medication abuse (4-5% of reported cases) which is the excess of

---

[78] Ahou Clémentine TANOH, op cit.

In addition, it is important to note the violation of the rights of the elderly and their active and passive neglect (authoritarian placement, confinement, etc.). In addition, it is necessary to note the violation of the rights of the elderly and their active neglect (authoritarian placement, confinement...) and passive neglect (forgetfulness, self neglect). [79]

In a partial way we can say that in the families that have in their bosom people of third age, these last ones undergo mistreatments of the psychological type, physical but to a different degree and it depends from a family to another. The most frequent of these abuses are located in the financial field from the institutions or elsewhere.

Regarding decision making within the family, the majority of respondents (72.3%) affirmed that they were consulted when taking care of their respective families, against 27.7% who denied or said the opposite. Let's note that among the respondents who affirmed that they are consulted before the decision is taken within their respective families, almost half or 43.2% say that they are consulted some of the time, 24.5% are consulted totally, those who are consulted partially occupy 19.6% against 12.7% who say that it is not totally. But for the respondents who denied being consulted within their families when making decisions, more than half (56.4%) put forward a reason of being neglected by the family, 30.8% say that they are considered as a child within the family. Likewise, 10.3% said that they were not considered because of their advanced age and 2.6% gave the reason that they did not stay with the family.

In part, it is worth noting that the opinion of the elder in the decision-making process in the family counts and weighs more, but this depends of course on the family.

As for the occupation of the elderly in the Goma health zone, most of the respondents (39.7%) were unemployed, 20.6% were retired, 14.2% were merchants, and 9.9% were government employees. However, 8.5% of the respondents practiced trades within their households and 7.1% practiced agriculture, so they were farmers.

The results of this study differ from those obtained by Maryse GAIMARD and Benoit LIBALI, who state that for the DRC, unlike in developed countries, the majority of the elderly population of the Congo is still active. More than half (52%) report being employed (49% of men and 54% of women). Retired persons, or those who have declared themselves as such, represent 17 percent of the population aged 60 or more; this proportion rises to 36 percent among the male population. In fact, women who do not declare

---

[79] Robert Hugonot and Françoise Busby quoted by Ahou Clémentine TANOH, op cit.

In the case of women who do not have a job, they say they are housewives (29%) and more rarely retired (3%). [80] In partial conclusion, let's say that pensions remain almost non-existent.

Indeed, the present study shows that out of the total number of respondents, 44 respondents (31.2%) contribute nothing throughout the month within their families, followed by 25 respondents (17.7%) who contribute more than $60 per month, 19 respondents (13.5%) who contribute less than $5 per month. But also, 18 respondents or 12.8% contribute in the range of 20 to 30$ per month within their respective families, 13 respondents or 9.2% contribute 6 to 10$ per month. However, those who contribute between $11 to $20 and $30 to $50 represent 11 respondents or 7.8%, so they are on the same level.

To finish this point, let's conclude in these words that the conditions of accommodation of the third age people are good, this taking into account the food security moderately assured, the consideration of their opinions in the taking of decisions within their respective families, the minimal degree of mistreatment of any field made to them within the families and elsewhere and/or institutions.

V.3. Housing needs experienced by seniors

If we consider the hypothesis according to which the premises adapted to their physical conditions, the desire to live in a home, and the need to protect their integuments would be housing needs experienced by the elderly in the health zone of Goma, the results of this study show that out of 141 respondents, more than half, or 58%, live in a house made of durable materials, followed by those who live in houses made of planks, or 54.6%, against a minority, or 2.8% and 1.4%, who live in houses made of tarpaulin and straw. In the same way, it appears that more than half, i.e. 53.9% of the respondents, say that the house they live in allows them to exercise all the physical movement against 46.1% who say the opposite. Among the respondents who denied that the house does not allow them to exercise all the physical movements, more than half of them, 66.1%, said that their houses do not have adequate chairs and armchairs, 16.9% mentioned the dampness (cold), 7.7% said that it is because there is no light in the house (electricity), while 6.2% mentioned the smallness of the house, and finally, 3.1% said that the stairs in the house are very long. Likewise, more than half, 63.8%, affirm that their houses are served with drinking water and electricity, while 36.2% prove the opposite opinion.

The above results diverge from those obtained by Esther Chrystelle EYINGA DIMI in her study on the living conditions and vulnerability of the elderly in

---

[80] Maryse GAIMARD and Benoit LIBALI, op cit.

The study also shows that 91.8% of elderly people live in homes that they own, while 8.2% of them are faced with housing insecurity. However, when we look at their housing status, we see that 29.1% of them live in low-standard housing and 43.1% in traditional type housing (improved or simple). A small proportion, 6.2%, live in precarious housing. We also note that 45.3% of the elderly do not have access to clean water. [81]

But also by confronting these same results with those of Maryse GAIMARD and Benoit LIBALI we notice a difference according to which the houses of the elderly are made of breeze blocks (26%), fired bricks (19%), unfired bricks (19%), planks (12%) or clay (15%).

Speaking of water and electricity, we note that among those who said that their dwellings have water and electricity, the majority of respondents (71.1%) say that water and electricity arrive irregularly, while 28.9% say that this service is regular in their dwellings.

Regarding the latrines used, 43.3% use a simple pit or borehole latrine in their households, 33.3% use a septic tank latrine, while 15.6% use a tank latrine and 7.8% use only an open latrine.

These results are close to those of Esther Chrystelle EYINGA DIMI, which show that more than 80% of elderly households have access to a source of drinking water: 22% of the elderly have a tap in the plot, 17% a tap outside the plot, 18% a well or borehole and 26% a spring. There are no disparities in the source of drinking water by gender of the heads of household or between elderly households and all households. [82]

However, Maryse GAIMARD and Benoit LIBALI say that nearly 20% of elderly households do not have a toilet in their home. The most common type of toilet is a latrine in the plot (63%). In addition, 16% of the elderly do not have a toilet and relieve themselves in the open. 12% have a modern toilet (4% in the dwelling and 8% in the plot) and 8% have a pit that can be emptied, slightly more often among the male population. Here again, the elderly are less well equipped than the general population, no doubt because they live in more rural areas and are less often equipped with a toilet.

---

[81] Esther Chrystelle EYINGA DIMI
[82] Esther Chrystelle EYINGA DIMI, op cit.

of modern toilets and where latrines in the plot and the use of nature (33%) are still widespread. [83]

The results of the same study show that more than half of the respondents, 57.4%, said that they wanted to live in the home, while 42.6% did not want to live in the home for the rest of their lives. Among the respondents who said that they would like to live in a nursing home, most of them (34.6%) said that the nursing home would be a place of rest for them, 33.3% said that they would meet their peers, 16.1% said that it would be a relief for their family, 12.3% said that they would feel safer and 3.7% said that they would be well cared for there. However, for those who do not wish to live in the home, more than half of them, 53.3%, give a reason to say that it is a lot for their children, 31.7% of them say that it is not their culture, while 8.3% say that it is a place of development that is not their culture, and finally, 6.7% consider it as an abandonment of the family. It is important to note that more than half of the respondents (61%) say that they want to live in conditions far from noise for the rest of their lives, 17.1% want to live in houses without excessive cold, 9.9% want to live in houses that are not flooded in rainy weather, while 6.4% want to live in a place where they will have more security and peace, and finally, 5.7% want to live far from illegal dumps that pollute the environment.

In conclusion, let us note at this point that the old people talk about accepting to live in a specialized institution. They could rest there; they would feel safer there; they would be cared for; it would relieve their family; they would meet people of their own age; they would like regular visits from their family. Hence the conditions said to be partially precarious.

[83] Maryse GAIMARD and Benoit LIBALI, op cit.

V.4. Types of housing referrals expressed by seniors

In testing the hypothesis that social assistance, family assistance, psychological support, medical care, and economic assistance through IGAs would be the types of referrals expressed by the elderly in the Goma health zone, the results of this study show that more than half (53.9%) have already benefited from external social assistance, compared to 46.1% who have never benefited from it. Among those who had received social assistance, most respondents (36.9%) said that they had received it from a church, 29.2% from an NGO, 15.5% from their previous place of work, 10.8% from the state, and 7.7% from family members. However, of those who said they had already received social assistance, more than half (55.4%) said that this assistance was for social support, 15.4% said it was for food, 12.3% had received a hut, while 10.8% had received practical advice, while 4.6% had received bonuses from their previous place of work and 1.5% spoke of counseling sessions. On the other hand, for those respondents who never received social assistance, a large majority, 89.5%, would like to receive it even though they did not have the chance to do so, compared to 10.5% who did not.

Regarding family support, this study shows that a large proportion (94.3%) of respondents want to receive support from their families, while a minority (5.7%) do not. However, among those who said they wanted family support, half (50.8%) wanted regular visits from their families while 49.2% wanted their basic needs met. For those who deny that they want family support, more than half, 66.7%, say that they do not want to cause their families to suffer, while 22.2% say that they are moving towards the end of their lives, while 11.1% say that they are self-sufficient.

Compared to the results of other authors, these results are almost similar to those of Nicole CAMPUIS LUCCIANI et al, who state that the vast majority of Senegalese respondents feel they can count on someone in case of a hard time, regardless of where they live. The same is true for Moroccans, except when they live in France where they feel little support; 65% of them feel they can only count on themselves or rely on God. [84]

Concerning the suffering of an illness, it appears from this study that a large majority, 97.2%, have already suffered from an illness during their daily life against a minority, 2.3%, who say they have never suffered from an illness. For those who said they had ever suffered from an illness, more than half (59.8%) had resorted to hospital treatment, 38% had resorted to self-medication and the use of medical plants, while 2.2% relied solely on prayer. However, a large majority (93.6%) of the respondents wanted specialized medical assistance in case of illness, while a minority (6.4%) did not.

If we consider the opinions expressed by the elderly on this point, we can partially conclude that they wish to live in retirement homes while offering them an opportunity to partially visit their respective families.

[84] Nicole CAMPUIS LUCCIANI et al, op cit.

Chapter Six:
CONCLUSION AND RECOMMENDATIONS
VI . 1. conclusion

At the end of this work entitled "Study on the needs of the establishment of homes for the elderly experienced by the elderly in the health zone of Goma" we wanted to know what are the needs of the establishment of homes for the elderly experienced by the elderly in the health zone of Goma. From this important constant, three specific questions followed:

> What are the housing conditions for the elderly in the Goma health zone?
> What are the housing needs of the elderly in the Goma health zone?
> What are the types of housing orientations expressed by the elderly in the Goma health zone?

Based on these questions we have formulated the following anticipated answers:

- S Food insecurity, psycho-physical abuse, lack of respect within their families, low financial contribution would be the conditions of accommodation of the elderly in the health zone of Goma;
- S Premises adapted to their physical conditions, the desire to live in the home, the need to protect their integuments would be housing needs experienced by the elderly in the health zone of Goma;
- S Social assistance, family assistance, psychological support, medical care, economic assistance through IGAs would be the types of orientations expressed by the elderly in terms of housing in the health zone of Goma.

In the search for an answer to these questions, we set out to achieve the general objective of identifying the needs for the establishment of old people's homes for the elderly in the health zone of Goma. The pursuit of this objective led us to operationalize it into the following four specific objectives:

> Determine the housing conditions for the elderly in the health zone of Goma;
> Identify the housing needs experienced by the elderly in the health zone of Goma;
> Determine the types of housing orientations expressed by the elderly in the Goma health zone.

This study is both evaluative and cross-sectional, and used both quantitative and qualitative data. The sample size for this study consisted of 141 older adults who fall within the age range of 65 years to 84 years and older. The data was collected by means of a survey questionnaire administered to 141 elderly people. It was also necessary to use an unstructured interview technique with a supporting interview guide to facilitate the collection of qualitative information from three household heads in the Goma health zone. Quantitative data were processed and analyzed in Microsoft Word and SPSS (Statistical Package of Social Sciences) software under Windows, and qualitative data were analyzed manually to test the hypotheses and arrive at the final results. After analyzing, processing, analyzing and interpreting the data, we reached the following conclusions:

Regarding living conditions, more than half of the respondents live in good conditions. If we look at the results of the score table, which show that out of **141** elderly people in the Goma health zone, **88** respondents (**62.4%**) answered positively to the criteria of good housing conditions, while **53** respondents (**37.6%**) indicated that the housing conditions were poor. Based on the above scores, we can conclude that the housing conditions for the elderly in the Goma Health Zone are ***good***. From this, we refute the hypothesis that food insecurity, psycho-physical mistreatment, low esteem within their families, and low financial contribution would be the housing conditions of the elderly in the Goma health zone;

When trying to identify the housing needs experienced by the elderly, it emerges that more than half of the respondents say that the house they live in allows them to exercise all the physical movements, against less than 1/4 who say the opposite. Among the respondents who denied that the house does not allow them to exercise all the physical movements, more than half either say that their houses do not have armchairs or adequate chairs, less than 1/3 talk about the humidity (cold), and the minority advance the reason that it is because in the house there is no light (current). In addition, speaking about water and electricity, more than half of the respondents affirm that their houses have drinking water and electricity, while most of them prove the opposite opinion, and among those who affirmed that their houses have water and electricity, a majority of the respondents say that the water and electricity arrive in an irregular way. If we look at the results of the score table, we see that out of **141** elderly people in the Goma health zone, **76** respondents (**54%**) answered positively to the criteria of good housing conditions, while **65** respondents (**46%**) indicated that housing conditions were poor. Based on the above scores, we can conclude that the housing conditions of the elderly in the Goma Health Zone are ***quite good***. Hence, we assert the hypothesis that the housing needs of the elderly in the Goma Health Zone are the need for a place to live that is adapted to their physical condition, the desire to live in a home, and the need to protect their skin;

Regarding the types of orientations expressed by the third age people regarding housing, the present study shows that a large proportion of respondents have the wish to have help from their respective families against a minority that does not. Drawing particular attention to the desire for medical assistance and the fact of having already suffered from an illness, we notice that a large majority of those who said they had already suffered from an illness also expressed the desire for medical assistance, while only a minority of those who had suffered from an illness did not express this desire. If we look at the results of the score table, we see that out of a total of **141** elderly people in the Goma health zone, **103** respondents (**73%**) answered favorably to the criteria for the types of referrals that are good, while **38** respondents (**27%**) **answered** the opposite. Based on the above scores, we can conclude that the types of referrals among the elderly in the Goma Health Zone are *good and they want to stay in the home for the rest of their lives.* From this, we assert the hypothesis that social assistance, family assistance, psychological support, medical care, and economic assistance through IGAs are the types of housing orientations expressed by the elderly in the Goma Health Zone.

VI.2 Recommendations

Taking into account the results and conclusions of this work, we suggest the following:

To the government

> That it strengthens the social security system throughout the national territory and gives all former workers in both the private and public sectors access to a pension;

> That it supports the organizations and associations that have in their midst initiatives of care or support of any kind for the elderly.

To the person in charge of the elderly in the health zone of Goma

> That they respond to the needs of economic, social, medical and health assistance.

To future researchers

Let them continue to address the topics with the same constituency as ours or even to approach this issue from the perspective of a feasibility study for the establishment of a home or nursing home, something we have not done; because we hope to have set the milestone and opened a large breach in a great site that is research in order to build a huge edifice that is science.

BIBLIOGRAPHY

1. Works
- Béatrice CARRAZ, *L'alimentation des personnes âgées*, Paris 2001.
- KARSTEN Thormaehlen, *aging and quality of life*, Ghana, 2012.
- Nicole CAMPUIS LUCCIANI et al, Aging population in southern countries: *Perception of the care of the elderly of Lebanese, Moroccan and Senegalese*, Article, University of Cheikh Anta Diope, Senegal, March 2011.
- Ms. Molopo, The *Need for a Law to Protect the Elderly in the DRC*, 2012.

2. Course
- KAMBALE KARAFULI Léopold, *public health course*, (unpublished), ULPGL/GOMA, G1FSDC, 2013-2014.
- NTABE NAMEGABE Edmond, *action research course,* (unpublished), ULPGL/GOMA ,2013-2014.

3. Memories and TFC
- Ahou Clémentine TANOH, *Etude sur les conditions de vie des personnes âgées en côte d'Ivoire*: Regard sur la maltraitance à Adjame Village, université de COCODY, (unpublished), Thèse, Abidjan 2006-2007.
- Bertrand Alain, *Hébergement des personnes âgées en famille d'accueil*, dissertation (unpublished), Institut supérieur de formation en soins infirmiers de Verdun, 1995-1998.
- Ira Bruno, *Conditions de vie des personnes âgées et solidarité sociale et familiale à l'épreuve de la pauvreté en milieu urbain, (unpublished),* Thesis, Abidjan 2007.
- Marcel NKOMA, *La sécurité sociale des personnes âgées en question*, in Workshop with the Ministry of Economy, Planning and Territorial Development, Cameroon, 2011.
- MUMBERE MUHASA Charmant, *problematic of the socio-economic situation of the elderly in the city of Goma*, Dissertation (unpublished), ISDR GL, 2012.
- OUAHIBA Benalla et al, La vieillesse au sud, approches comparatives, *Quelle est la place des personnes de troisièmes âges en perte d'autonomie*, Article, University of Bouira, Algeria, March 2011.

4. **Reports and articles**
   - *Goma* health zone central office, *annual report*, 2012-2013.
   - Bureau de l'état civil, commune de Goma, census report by age group, 2013.
   - Esther Chrystelle EYINGA DIMI, *Living conditions and vulnerability of the elderly in the South*, Socioeconomic situations of the elderly in Cameroon, art, Université Bordeaux Segalen, Centre Émile Durkheim - CEPED, March 2011.
   - Maryse GAIMARD and Benoit LIBALI, *Vieillissement et conditions de vie des personnes âgées en République du Congo*, art, Université Bordeaux Segalen, Centre Émile Durkheim - CEPED, France March 2011.
   - Ministry of Health, 2002.
   - Mohammed BEDROUNI: *Characteristics and conditions of social and health care of the elderly Moroccan and Algerian Ressemblances and dissimilarities* in the old age in the south comparative approach, Art, university of saad Daheleb of blida, Algeria, March 2011.
   - Mouftaou AMADOU SANNI, Population aging in southern countries: *Urban challenges of aging in Benin*, CEFORP, May 2011.
   - WHO, *Ghana takes care of its aging population*, October 2013.
   - HEAL PAGE Report: *Africa's Ageing Problem:* Summary, unpublished report, Nairobi, 2000.
   - WHO report, *Elder Abuse,* 2012.
   - WHO report, *aging and the life course*, 2012.
   - Valérie GOLAZ and Philippe ANTOINE, *Living conditions and vulnerability of the elderly in the South:* What are the elderly in a vulnerable situation, comparative study between Uganda and Senegal, art, France, March 2011.
   - Marcel NGOMBO, Interview with the provincial minister in charge of Public Health, Social Affairs, Solidarity and Family on the precarious living conditions at the TSHOPO home for the elderly.

5. **Dictionaries**
   - Dictionary, le robert de poche, paris, 2009.

6. **Webography**
   - http://www.who.int/features/factfiles/ageing/fr/, accessed March 22, 2014 at 9:20 a.m.; by KARSTEN Thormaehlen.
   - http://www.ceped.org/cdrom/meknes/spipcddf.htmParticle33, accessed May 17, 2014 at 1:30 p.m.; Marcel NKOMA, *The social security of the elderly in question.*
   - http://www.who.int/violenceinjury prevention, accessed March 24, 2014 at 11:15 a.m.; WHO Report, *Elder Abuse,* 2012.
   - http://www.who.int/ageing/projects/elder abuse/en/, accessed March 24, 2014 at 11:15 a.m.; WHO Report, *Aging and the Life Course*, 2012.

- http://www.who.int/features/2013/ghana-living-longer/fr/, accessed March 24, 2014 at 10:30 a.m.; WHO, *Ghana Takes Care of Its Aging Population*, October 2013.
- http://www.acpcongo.com/index.php?option=com_content&view=article&id=27837:rd-congo. Accessed May 17, 2014; Ms. Molopo, *Need for a law to protect the elderly in the DRC*, 2012.
- http://radiookapi.net/regions/province-orientale/2013/10/03/province-orientale-conditions-de-vie-precaire-au-home-des-vieillards-de-la-tshopo/#.U3fEOT_upK4, accessed May 17, 2014 at 1:30 p.m.; Marcel NGOMBO, *Interview with the provincial minister in charge of public health*.
- http://www.laprosperiteonline.net/show.php?id=13825&rubrique=Nation
- LA voix des sans - voix (VSV), *Rapport d'information sur les personnes âgées à Kinshasa/R.D.C*, July 1999, available at http://www.congonline.com/vsv/rapports/rapports1/07.htm.
- George MUSAVULI, Care for the elderly, assistance program, BUTEMBO, August 2011, available at http://www.congoforum.be/fr/nieuwsdetail.asp?subitem=3&newsid=179865&Actualiteit=selected, accessed March 24, 2014 at 10:30 am.
- WHO, Report on *elder abuse*, August 2011, available at http://www.who.int/mediacentre/factsheets/fs357/fr/.

APPENDI CES

LIBERAL UNIVERSITY OF THE GREAT LAKES COUNTRIES
FACULTY OF COMMUNITY HEALTH AND DEVELOPMENT
SURVEY QUESTIONNAIRE

With the elderly in the Goma health zone
My name is .... I am working on behalf of **SHUKURU KASIWA Benjamin**, a student in his second degree in Community Health and Development, Option: Management and Administration of Health Projects at ULPGL/GOMA. His objective is to evaluate the needs for the establishment of old people's homes in the health zone of Goma. For this purpose, your contribution through the answers to the questions we will ask you is of utmost importance. We guarantee that all answers will be kept anonymous and secret in all respects.

May I start please?
We thank you in advance
Instructions: Circle or box the true answer

N°	Questions	Codes/Answers	Go to
	I. Identification of the respondent		
Q1	Age of respondent	1. 65 - 69 years 2. 70- 74 years 3. 75- 79 years 4. 80-84 years 5. 85 years and older	
Q2	Gender of respondent	1. Male 2. Female	
Q3	What is your level of education?	1. Primary completed 2. Primary not completed 3. Secondary completed 4. Secondary not completed 5. university completed 6. University not completed 7. No level	
Q4	What religious denomination are you?	1. Catholic 2. Protestant 3. Muslim 4. Other.................	
Q5	What is your marital status?	1. Single 2. Married 3. Widow(er) 4. Divorced 5. United in fact 6. Other to specify	
	II. Housing conditions for the elderly		
Q6	What are the living conditions like in your household?	1. Very good 2. Good 3. Fairly good 4. Bad 5. very bad 6. Other to be specified.	
Q7	What food do you usually eat?	1. Cassava or corn fufu 2. Bean 3. Fish 4. Vegetables and fruits 5. Other to be specified....	
Q8	How often do you eat per day?	1. Once a day 2. Twice a day 3. Three times a day 4. More than three times/day	
Q9	Have you ever been physically abused in your family or elsewhere?	1. Yes 2. No	If not go to Q13
Q10	If so, which one?	1. Slap or blow 2. Harassment 3. Untreated or poorly treated pressure sores 4. brutality 5. deliberate injury 6. Other to be specified ...	
Q11	Have you ever been emotionally abused in your family or elsewhere?	1. Yes 2. No	If not go to Q116

Q12	If so, which one?	1. Insult 2. Shocking words 3. humiliation 4. I am stressed 5. Other to be specified ...	
Q13	Are you consulted when decisions are made within the family?	1. Yes 2. No	If no go to Q17
Q14	If so, are your views taken into account?	1. Not quite 2. Sometimes 3. Partially 4. Totally	
Q15	If not, why not?	1. I am not considered to be at fault for old age 2. I am neglected 3. I am considered a child 4. Other to be specified ...	
Q16	What is your profession?	1. Trader 2. State employee 3. Cultivator 4. Retired 5. Unemployed 6. Other to be specified	
Q17	How much can you estimate your contribution to your monthly household income?	1. Less than $5 2. 6 à 10$ 3. 11 à 20$ 4. 21 à 30$ 5. 30 à 50$ 6. More than $60 7. No income	
		III. Housing needs experienced by the elderly	
Q18	What type of housing do you live in?	1. Durable material 2. Plank house 3. Tarpaulin house 4. Other to be specified.................	
Q19	Does the house you live in allow for all physical movement?	1. Yes 2. No	If yes go to Q23
Q20	If not, how?	1. No armchairs or adequate chairs 2. The stairs are very long 3. humidity (cold) 4. no light 5. Other to be specified.................	
Q21	Is your home served by water and electricity?	1. Yes 2. No	If no go to Q17
Q22	If so, how often?	1. Regularly 2. Irregularly	
Q23	What type of latrine do you use?	1. Single pit latrine 2. Septic tank latrine 3. Latrine with tank 4. Other to be specified......	
Q24	How often is your latrine maintained?	1. once/s 2. Twice/s 3. Three times/s 4. Four times/s 5. More than five times/s 6. No time	
Q25	Have you ever heard of an old people's home?	1. Yes 2. No	
Q26	Would you like to live in a retirement home for the rest of your life?	1. Yes 2. No	If not go to Q30
Q27	If so, why?	1. I will be able to rest there 2. I will feel safer there 3. I will be well cared for there 4. My family will be relieved 5. I'll be with people my own age; 6. Other to specify.............	
Q28	If not, why not?	1. I rely heavily on my children 2. This would be an abandonment 3. It's not a place of fulfillment 4. It is not in our culture 5. My family can help me 6. Other to specify.............	

Q29	What conditions do you want to live in for the rest of your life?	1. Away from the noise 2. In dwellings not flooded during rainy weather 3. Housing far from the illegal dumps that pollute the environment 4. House without excessive cold 5. Other	
	IV. Types of orientations expressed by the elderly		
Q30	Have you ever been a recipient of outside social assistance?	1. Yes 2. No	If no go to Q35
Q31	If so, where does it come from?	1. NGO 2. The State 3. Church 4. At my previous place of work 5. Other to be specified	
Q32	If so, what was it about?	1. Social framing 2. Practical advice 3. Counselling session 4. Other	
Q33	If not, would you still like to have some?	1. Yes 2. No	
Q34	Would you like help from your family?	1. Yes 2. No	If not go to Q38
Q35	If so, how?	1. I would like my family to visit me regularly 2. By meeting my basic needs 3. Other to report	
Q36	If not, why not?	1. I am self-sufficient 2. I tend to the end of my life 3. I don't want to suffer family 4. Other to specify........................	
Q37	Have you ever suffered from an illness?	1. Yes 2. No	If not go to Q41
Q38	If so, how were you treated?	1. Self-medication / use of traditional medicinal plants 2. I went to the hospital 3. Other to specify	
Q39	Would you like special medical assistance in case of illness?	1. Yes 2. No	
Q40	Do you have a desire to receive economic assistance to support yourself?	1. Yes 2. No	
Q41	If so, what type?	1. In kind 2. In cash 3. By an IGA 4. Other to specify...	

Thank you for your answers.

LIBERAL UNIVERSITY OF THE GREAT LAKES COUNTRIES
FACULTY OF COMMUNITY HEALTH AND DEVELOPMENT

Interview Guide

With the people in charge of the households of the elderly in the health zone of Goma, particularly in the KYSHERO and LES VOLCANS districts.

My name is **SHUKURU KASIWA Benjamin**, a student in my second degree in Community Health and Development, Option: Management and Administration of Health Projects at ULPGL/GOMA. My objective is to evaluate the needs for the establishment of old people's homes in the health zone of Goma. For this, your contribution through opinions on this subject is of utmost importance. We guarantee that all answers will be kept anonymous and secret in all respects.

We thank you in advance

01. According to you, what are the conditions under which you house the old man in your household?

02. What are the housing needs experienced by the elderly in your household

03. What types of referrals are expressed by the elderly in your household

Thank you for the opinions

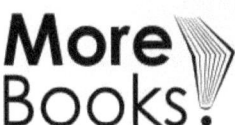 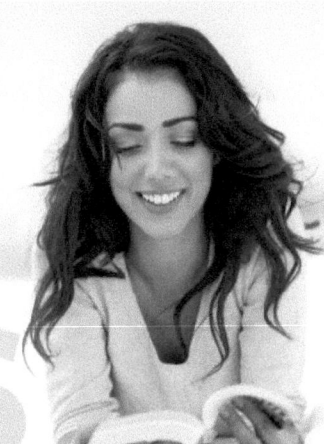

I want morebooks!

Buy your books fast and straightforward online - at one of world's fastest growing online book stores! Environmentally sound due to Print-on-Demand technologies.

Buy your books online at
www.morebooks.shop

Kaufen Sie Ihre Bücher schnell und unkompliziert online – auf einer der am schnellsten wachsenden Buchhandelsplattformen weltweit! Dank Print-On-Demand umwelt- und ressourcenschonend produziert.

Bücher schneller online kaufen
www.morebooks.shop

 info@omniscriptum.com
www.omniscriptum.com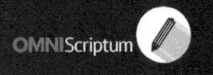

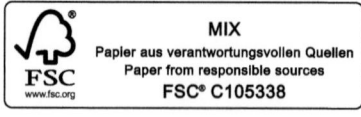

Printed by Books on Demand GmbH, Norderstedt / Germany